Your Personal Guide to Living Well with Fibromyalgia

Your Personal Guide to Living Well with Fibromyalgia

AN OFFICIAL PUBLICATION OF THE ARTHRITIS FOUNDATION
Atlanta, Georgia

LONGSTREET PRESS, INC.
Atlanta, Georgia

Published by
LONGSTREET PRESS, INC.
A subsidiary of Cox Newspapers,
A subsidiary of Cox Enterprises, Inc.
2140 Newmarket Parkway
Suite 122
Marietta, GA 30067

Printed in the United States of America
1st printing 1997

Library of Congress Card Catalog Number: 96-79811

ISBN: 1-56352-382-5

Table of Contents

Foreword

Fibromyalgia is a common condition characterized by muscular pain, fatigue, and poor sleep. Because this condition is difficult to diagnose, you may find yourself undergoing needless laboratory tests and X-rays, which only add frustration and a big medical bill to the pain and other symptoms that brought you to the doctor in the first place. Some doctors may even say, "You look good, the laboratory tests are normal, and nothing is wrong with you. Perhaps you are just imagining this pain." Neither scenario should occur. Knowledgeable physicians can recognize and diagnose fibromyalgia, and they can recommend an effective management approach to help control the symptoms.

You, the patient, are the central figure in this management process. You must take the initiative, and the first step is learning. The simple process of understanding fibromyalgia will eliminate the fear of the unknown. You will come to realize that although the condition is painful, it is neither crippling nor necessarily progressive. More importantly, you will learn that you can control your fibromyalgia, with exercise and a variety of pain- and fatigue-management strategies. This book will give you the information you need to succeed.

DOYT L. CONN, MD
Senior Vice President of Medical Affairs
Arthritis Foundation, Atlanta, GA

Acknowledgments

Your Personal Guide To Living Well With Fibromyalgia is written for people who have fibromyalgia and their family and friends. Much of the book was adapted from the participant's manual of the Arthritis Foundation's Fibromyalgia Self-Help Course, a program developed in the late 1980s and originally supported by the Norma Borie Fibromyalgia Research and Education Program Fund. After successful implementation by its Southern California chapter, the National Office of the Arthritis Foundation proceeded with a national pilot test of this course and began offering it through Arthritis Foundation chapters in 1995.

Many volunteers and staff contributed to the development of the Fibromyalgia Self-Help Course, including Dorothy Anderle Johnson; Carol Beardmore, PhD; Peng Thim Fan, MD; Fran Goldfar; Mary Ellen Kullman; Kenneth Nies, MD; Lori Odendahl; Marilyn Potts; Stuart Silverman, MD; and Dena Slonaker.

Individuals who field tested and/or provided critiques to make the course appropriate for national distribution include: Teresa Brady, Wendy McBrair, Lila Roseman, Nella Schnaufer, and members of the National Patient and Community Services Program subcommittee.

Many of the materials contained in this manual were adapted from the Arthritis Self-Help Course or the Chronic Disease Self-Management Course developed by Kate Lorig, RN, DrPH, and her colleagues at the Stanford Arthritis Center. The significant contributions of individuals involved in the development, evaluation and ongoing implementation of these programs are deeply appreciated.

Your Personal Guide To Living Well With Fibromyalgia is not meant to take the place of treatment and teaching provide by a doctor and other health-care professionals. However, it should help you understand your condition so you can take an active role in keeping it under control.

Special thanks to the following individuals who reviewed this book: Walter G. Barr, MD, Rheumatology, Loyola University, Maywood, Illinois.; Robert M. Bennett, MD, University of Oregon School of Medicine, Portland; Mary Brown, S.Surrey, British Columbia; Pat Harrington, Wisconsin Dells, Wisconsin.; Dorothy A. Johnson, DNSC, FNP, University of Southern California Medical Center, Los Angeles; Marian Minor, PhD, PT, University of Missouri, Columbia; Judy Conley, Lansing, Michigan.

If you have any questions as you read the book, write them down and contact your local Arthritis Foundation chapter or take the list with you to your doctor.

CREDITS:
Publisher: Longstreet Press
Editorial Director: Adrienne Greer
Art Director: Jennifer Rogers
Cover Design: Jennifer Rogers
Illustrator: Shawn Carson
Designer: Audrey Graham
Writers: Doyt Conn, MD, Adrienne Greer, Krista Reese, Dianne
  Witter, Jane Zanca
Copyeditor: Krista Reese

ARTHRITIS FOUNDATION REVIEWERS:
Janet Austin, PhD, Vice President of the American Juvenile Arthritis
  Organization (AJAO) and Special Groups
Michele Boutaugh, BSN, MPH, Vice President of Patient and
  Community Services
Doyt L. Conn, MD, Senior Vice President of Medical Affairs
Leigh DeLozier, Director of Consumer Publications
Cindy McDaniel, Vice President of Publications
Susan Percy, Managing Editor, *Arthritis Today*

Introduction

The more you know about fibromyalgia, the better you'll be at managing it. The first section of this book is designed to educate. Chapter 1 provides a complete history of the condition, from the medical profession's earliest official diagnoses to the most recent researchers' findings. Chapter 2 lays out the wide array of treatments, from established to experimental.

Part Two moves from education to action, beginning with your role: captain of your fate and manager of your condition. This section helps you establish goals and provides tips and exercises for reaching them, from dealing with your doctor to deciding what's important to you.

Part Three offers practical self-help for the most common symptoms of fibromyalgia: pain, fatigue, and fitful sleep. Guidelines are also provided to help you recognize and overcome mental obstacles like anxiety, grief, and depression about your physical condition.

Equally important are proactive approaches to living well. Part Four presents tips on diet, exercise, and emotional health, created especially for people with fibromyalgia.

Throughout the book, you'll find a number of activities and exercises, designed to prompt new ways of thinking about and managing your condition. Try as many as you like, and keep only the methods that work best for you.

Fibromyalgia can't be cured by pills or surgery. But you can get better. It all begins with a commitment to doing all you can to help yourself. Consider this book your resource, your companion, and your guide in the journey toward a healthy life with fibromyalgia.

Your Personal Guide to Living Well with Fibromyalgia

PART ONE

Fibromyalgia: A Primer

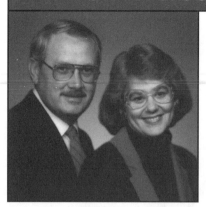

Ann with her husband, Allan

Life on the Seesaw of Chronic Pain
by Ann B. McPherson
Kill Devil Hills, NC

At the tender age of 30, I had surgery for a ruptured disc in my lower back. From that point on I had bouts of pain that came and went pretty much like the weather. Ten years and several surgeries later, a neurologist diagnosed me with fibromyalgia. It was nice finally to know what was wrong with my body. He explained a lot of the crazy symptoms I'd been experiencing over the years, but to my dismay, he couldn't give me the information that I desperately needed for my peace of mind. Thus began my search for anything and everything I could find on the topic.

My search started with a phone call to the Arthritis Foundation. Eventually I learned about a book by a psychiatrist with fibromyalgia, and began collecting a few newsletters on the condition. I have sought help through books on relaxation and learning to cope with chronic pain. I'm a firm believer in knowing what is wrong and learning all you can about your problem. For me, education and an exercise regimen of walking and stretching, in conjunction with the right medicines, have been my keys to getting as much of my health back as possible. Yes, there are still days I can hardly walk across the floor, but all I have to do is remember where I was, and how far I've come. That's enough to keep anyone on the upswing of that ever-moving seesaw.

CHAPTER 1

History and Background

What Is Fibromyalgia?

The official definition—and precise naming—of fibromyalgia is a relatively recent event, despite the fact that its symptoms have been discussed in medical literature since the early 1900s. The medical community's recognition of fibromyalgia slowly increased in the early 1980s, as some doctors began developing treatments for the condition. In 1989, the highly respected *Textbook on Rheumatology* included a chapter on "fibrositis" in its third edition. But the author of the chapter, Robert M. Bennett, MD, professor of medicine and director of the division of arthritis and rheumatic diseases at the Oregon Health Sciences University in Portland, pointed out that the name didn't really fit. Literally defined, fibrositis meant inflammation (Latin "itis") of fibrous tissue (Latin "fibro"). A year later, a criteria committee at the American College of Rheumatology (ACR), including Dr. Bennett, agreed that the condition should more appropriately be called fibromyalgia syndrome—pain (Greek "algia") of the muscle (Greek "mys") and fibrous tissue (Latin "fibro").

The ACR (the professional association of rheumatologists) also released its criteria for diagnosis, a list of classic symptoms of the syndrome:

- history of widespread pain (on both sides of the body, above and below the waist, present for at least three months)
- pain in at least 11 of 18 "tender point" sites

Tender points are areas of the body that are painful when pressed. People with fibromyalgia may have tender points in several places, including the base of the skull, above and between the shoulder blades, below the elbows, in the lower back, on the hips, and behind the knees (see diagram, page 4).

These tender areas are similar in location to sore and tender areas in other common muscle and muscle-attachment disorders, such as tennis elbow and trochanteric bursitis (irritation of the trochanteric muscle attachments outside the hip). They are almost always on both sides of the body. Sometimes tender sites can go unnoticed until a doctor, or other trained specialist who knows exactly where to press, applies pressure.

Not all physicians are familiar with the evaluation of tender points, but most rheumatologists (specialists in arthritis and rheumatic diseases) know how to perform such an examination. Fibromyalgia is considered to be an arthritis-related condition, but unlike arthritis, it does not damage joints. *Soft-tissue rheumatism* is a broad term to include disorders causing pain and stiffness around the joints, and in muscles and bones. Because its symptoms occur in muscles and joints, fibromyalgia is included in this group of disorders.

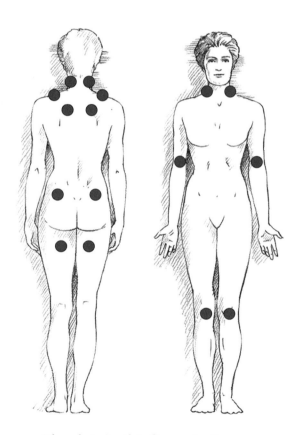

The dots in this figure indicate tender points. Pain in these points is the most distinctive characteristic of fibromyalgia.

Some Common Symptoms in Adults

No two people with fibromyalgia experience exactly the same symptoms to exactly the same degree, and the symptoms in children (see page 7) may differ somewhat from those of adults.

Pain

Muscle pain is the most prominent and common symptom of fibromyalgia. It is generally felt all over, although it may start in one region, such as the neck and shoulders, and spread over a period of time. Pain may be very intense in one area and then disappear, only to appear in another area. Although pain may occur around the joints, the joints themselves are not involved.

Some people with fibromyalgia describe their pain as knifelike in intensity; others compare it to an all-over muscle cramp. The pain can vary according to the time of day, activity level, weather, individual sleep patterns, and stress. Most people with fibromyalgia say that some degree of pain is always present, and many say it feels like a persistent flu. For some, the pain is quite severe.

Fatigue and Sleep Disturbance

About 90 percent of people with fibromyalgia report moderate or severe fatigue. In fact, scientific studies have demonstrated that most people with fibromyalgia have abnormal sleep patterns—they may find it hard to fall asleep, and wake up frequently once they do. They often wake up feeling tired, even after sleeping through the night. The resulting fatigue can range from listlessness and decreased exercise endurance to exhaustion, varying during the day and from one day to the next. See Chapter 7 for more information on sleep.

Depression and Anxiety

Changes in mood and thinking are common, too. Many people with fibromyalgia report feeling "blue" or "down," although only about 25 percent are clinically depressed, requiring care of a mental-health professional such as a psychiatrist (see Chapter 9). Some people also feel anxious. Such feelings may be a result of fibromyalgia, or they may be a cause of it. However, some researchers feel there may be a biological link between fibromyalgia and some forms of depression and chronic anxiety.

People with fibromyalgia may report difficulty with concentration, short-term memory, or simple mental tasks. These symptoms are common in people with sleep disturbances of all kinds.

Other Signs and Symptoms

Headaches are common in fibromyalgia, especially muscular or tension headaches and migraine headaches. Bladder irritability and spasms, resulting in a frequent need to urinate, as well as irritable bowel syndrome, or alternating constipation and diarrhea, can also be problematic. Skin may temporarily change color because of circulatory sensitivity to temperature and moisture. The hands, arms, feet, legs, or face can tingle or become numb. New studies of people with fibromyalgia have reported other symptoms, including problems with the temporomandibular joint (TMJ, in which the jaws hinge), cramps, dizziness, and abdominal pain. These symptoms can come and go, and may become worse during times of illness, stress, or excessive physical exertion.

SOME POTENTIAL SYMPTOMS

- Generalized pain
- Fatigue
- Insomnia
- Headaches
- Morning stiffness
- Irritable bowel syndrome
- Bladder irritability
- Numbness and tingling in extremities
- Circulatory problems
- Nonrestorative sleep
- Cold intolerance

Who Gets Fibromyalgia?

According to unpublished data from the National Arthritis Data Workgroup, some 3.7 million Americans have fibromyalgia, making it one of the most common types of pain syndromes. It occurs most often in people between the ages of 20 and 55, though it can affect anyone, including children. Women are 10 times more likely than men to have it.

Men or women with other rheumatic diseases such as rheumatoid arthritis (RA, a chronic, inflammatory autoimmune disease involving the joints, and causing pain, swelling, and deformity) and lupus (an inflammatory connective tissue autoimmune disease that can involve the skin, joints, kidneys, blood, and other organs and is associated with anti-nuclear antibodies) are at greater risk of having fibromyalgia, with about 20 percent of those with RA developing the condition. Fibromyalgia is the second most common disorder seen by rheumatologists. No one knows exactly why people with RA are prone to fibromyalgia. However, there does not seem to be a cause-and-effect relationship between the two conditions—generally, when RA improves, fibromyalgia is unaffected. Fibromyalgia sometimes occurs in more than one member of the same family, but doctors have not verified a hereditary link or genetic type common among people with the syndrome. The fact that it sometimes appears within families could be simply because it's a common condition.

Children and Fibromyalgia

Although fibromyalgia is most common in women, the disorder has become increasingly common in adolescents. In fact, musculoskeletal pain syndromes represent the most common problems seen by pediatric rheumatologists. Of children with chronic pain syndromes, 25 percent to 40 percent fulfill the criteria for juvenile fibromyalgia syndrome.

The syndrome was first reported in the medical literature in 1985 by Muhammed B. Yunus, MD, of the University of Illinois College of Medicine. Many of the symptoms seen by Dr. Yunus's group were similar to those seen in adults with fibromyalgia, but the children had fewer tender points (see tender points diagram earlier in this chapter). Because the American College of Rheumatology has developed diagnostic criteria for adults, the validity for this criteria in the pediatric population is still unknown.

Up to 28 percent of adults with fibromyalgia report the onset of symptoms during childhood. The Yunus study of 33 children with fibromyalgia identified the following symptoms:

- generalized aches and pains
- stiffness
- morning fatigue
- chronic headaches
- irritable bowel syndrome

According to the *Primer on the Rheumatic Diseases, 10th Ed.,* children with fibromyalgia, like adults, often sleep poorly. The study by Dr. Yunus also cites noisy surroundings, poor sleep, and significant family dysfunction and depression among children with the syndrome.

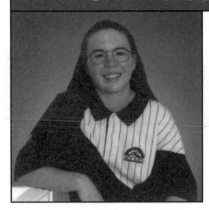

Keep Your Face to the Sunshine
by Stephanie R. Nelson
Sterling, CO

When I was a sophomore in high school, my life changed drastically. I had played volleyball competitively since seventh grade, but constant chest pain forced me to quit playing during the middle of the season that year. After a year of going to cardiologists, physical therapists, osteopaths and homeopaths, I was diagnosed with fibromyalgia and rheumatoid arthritis by my rheumatologist.

Although my diagnosis came as a relief, there was also a sense of anger, loss and hopelessness. In the 18 months since my diagnosis, I have learned a great deal about my condition and myself. A favorite quote that has helped me reads: "Keep your face to the sunshine and you cannot see the shadows."

It is weakening to live in the shadows. I have been there many times, and it takes great effort to get out of this state of mind. When I am having a bad day, it helps tremendously to do things that I enjoy. I can often find the sunshine again when I am with my friends. I don't think I would have been able to survive without concentrating on attitude, something I focus on almost every hour of every day. Because exercise and stretching are crucial to how I feel, I lift weights, run, walk and ride my bike. Even if I am feeling tired, walking a few minutes helps me both physically and mentally.

I try to value each day that I feel good enough to go to school, exercise and everything else people my age do. It is really hard to see my classmates participating in sports while I am up in the stands watching, or on the sidelines taking photographs for our yearbook. But I will not be discouraged!

My classmates have been supportive through my ups and downs. I don't like having a lot of attention, and they honor this. When I am at school, I try to concentrate on school only. I don't want to think about the difference that exists between my friends and me, but subconsciously I am always aware of that. My friends give me hope and make me realize the importance of having a support system.

I know that by looking ahead with a positive attitude, even while realizing my limitations, I can handle all the curves my life may throw. Even though it's difficult sometimes, I keep my face to the sunshine.

The Diagnosis Dilemma

No evidence of fibromyalgia appears on X-rays or through laboratory tests; nor is there a diagnostic "marker" in the blood. People with fibromyalgia often look healthy, with no outward signs of pain or fatigue. Diagnosis of children may be especially difficult because they often have trouble describing their symptoms.

Diagnosis may depend both on the identification of symptoms and on the exclusion of other possible conditions. Lab tests can rule out maladies with similar symptoms, including hypothyroidism and hyperparathyroidism. However, if you have widespread pain plus tender points, your diagnosis is likely to be fibromyalgia syndrome, even if you have another condition.

Despite its prevalence, fibromyalgia remains unfamiliar to most people. Many doctors weren't taught about the condition, because medical schools began teaching about it only relatively recently. That lack of general knowledge, along with the lack of objective physical evidence for the syndrome from X-rays or lab tests, is what leads many on a long and often frustrating quest for answers.

According to Don L. Goldenberg, MD, chief of rheumatology and director of the Arthritis-Fibromyalgia Center at Newton-Wellesley Hospital in Newton, Massachusetts, studies show that it takes most people with fibromyalgia an average of five years after they start experiencing symptoms to find a diagnosis. That means five years of sanity-testing frustration added to fibromyalgia's chronic symptoms.

Fortunately, there is now a greater understanding of fibromyalgia among the medical community. Although the underlying cause remains undetermined, new research has uncovered exciting leads and better treatments.

What Causes Fibromyalgia?

Scientists have not positively established any single cause for the disorder. Some researchers believe that an injury or trauma, physical or emotional, may affect the central nervous system's response to pain. Others believe an infection, such as a flu virus, may trigger fibromyalgia in susceptible people. Another group suspects that lack of exercise and changes in muscle metabolism may play a role, or that the opposite—muscle overuse—may be the key. There is an established link between fibromyalgia and depression, but no one knows if it's a cause of or effect of the ailment.

For years, a long-standing theory held that fibromyalgia may begin with a defect in how muscles use energy. However, in 1995, *Arthritis Today* magazine reported on a study, conducted at the Boston University School of Medicine and published in *Arthritis and Rheumatism*, that challenges that theory. Using new technology, rheumatologist Robert Simms, MD, associate professor of medicine and director of clinical rheumatology at Boston University School of Medicine, and his colleagues were able to show that muscle uses energy in much the same way among people who have equivalent levels of aerobic fitness, whether they have fibromyalgia or not.

Recent findings have supplied intriguing leads about the nature of the condition. For example, researchers are interested in similarities between fibromyalgia and chronic fatigue syndrome, another tenacious condition of unknown origin. (In the fourth edition of the *Textbook of Rheumatology*, Dr. Bennett titled one chapter, "The Fibromyalgia Syndrome: Myofascial Pain and the Chronic Fatigue Syndrome.")

One of the hottest areas of research into fibromyalgia's underlying cause is hormones. Secreted by glands, hormones are among the body's most powerful substances. Neural hormones are the chemical messengers of the central nervous system, affecting such functions as sleep, pain sensation, immunity, the constriction and dilation of blood vessels, and even emotions.

Somatomedin C

In 1992, Dr. Bennett and his colleagues found a possible clue to the nature of fibromyalgia, linking it to disturbed sleep. As described in the March/April 1993 issue of *Arthritis Today*, the body (specifically the liver and probably the kidney) secretes a growth hormone called somatomedin C. Essential to the body's task of rebuilding itself, somatomedin C is secreted only in stage-4 sleep, the deepest and most restorative level of the daily sleep period.

Dr. Bennett found that people with fibromyalgia had significantly lower blood levels of somatomedin C than those without the condition. However, more recent studies have failed to support that conclusion. One researcher with a special interest in this field is Harvey Moldofsky, MD, of the Center for Sleep and Chronobiology at Western Division Toronto Hospital. He and his co-workers, pioneers in the new science of chronobiology—the timing of biologic events—went on to show that when the same sleep abnormality that occurs in deep sleep (sleep stages 3 and 4) was induced in people without fibromyalgia, they too developed symptoms of the condition.

Serotonin and Substance P

Another hormone, serotonin, plays an important role in the central nervous system to reduce pain and facilitate sleep.

You might think of the central nervous system as a central electrical wiring system for the body. Like wires, neurons carry electrical impulses from the farthest reaches of fingers and toes to the spinal cord, where all the wiring comes together—as in your home's circuit-breaker box. And just as the electric company monitors your breaker box through wires, the brain manages the nervous system through spinal cord connections.

When the body is injured, neurons go to red alert, serving as a hot line and surveillance system. The news of the injury reaches the brain at lightning speed. A molecule called substance P is released in the neurons and in the spinal cord. Its job is to send a loud pain message back to the brain.

Fortunately, the body has a way of turning down the volume on the message—serotonin and other natural painkilling substances are released in the brain and spinal cord to do this job. Jon Russell, MD, PhD, assistant professor of medicine and director of the University Clinical Research Center at the University of Texas Health Sciences Center in San Antonio, is dedicated to understanding this function and its role in fibromyalgia.

"It should come as no surprise that abnormalities in the production or levels of [these] chemicals . . . in the spinal cord or brain would influence how much pain is perceived by the individual," he says.

Dr. Russell's research team found that serotonin may be low or poorly metabolized in people with fibromyalgia. This may be an important finding, because serotonin also facilitates deep, restorative sleep—the lack of which is a known culprit in fibromyalgia.

Studies have shown that levels of substance P in the spinal cord are elevated (about three times the normal level) in people with fibromyalgia, compared with people who do not have fibromyalgia. One recent study indicated that elevated levels of substance P were still high when a second sample of spinal fluid was drawn weeks to months later, indicating a persistent elevation. Also, applying painful pressure to tender points did not spur an increase in the level. The latter finding suggests that levels of substance P are increased in people with fibromyalgia due to an internal physiologic process, rather than in response to external stimuli such as bumps and bruises.

Researchers must await additional studies to confirm these findings before assigning a causative role to substance P or serotonin.

Fibromyalgia and Sexual Abuse

Researchers have questioned the possible link between physical and emotional trauma, such as sexual abuse, and fibromyalgia. In 1995, two studies were published in *Arthritis & Rheumatism* on the prevalence of sexual and physical abuse in women with fibromyalgia syndrome. In that same journal, James I. Hudson, MD, and Harrison G. Pope Jr., MD, published an editorial exploring whether or not childhood sexual abuse causes fibromyalgia.

Neither study concluded that sexual abuse causes fibromyalgia. Rather, there appeared to be an association between sexual abuse and the number and severity of associated symptoms related to fibromyalgia. However, both were retrospective studies in which characteristics were reviewed by looking into the patient's past. The editorial stressed "that even if there existed a true correlation between childhood sexual abuse and fibromyalgia, it is a fallacy to conclude that correlation demonstrates causality."

A prospective longitudinal study that is a forward-looking review is needed. Although a prospective study would be cumbersome and expensive, it is necessary to assess the relationship between emotional trauma and conditons like fibromyalgia.

HPA Hormones

Intrigued by patients' descriptions of when fibromyalgia first emerges and then recurs, Leslie Crofford, MD, assistant professor of internal medicine at the University of Michigan in Ann Arbor, is probing the meaning of stress in the fibromyalgia syndrome. "Since fibromyalgia often begins during periods of intense physical or emotional stress—and symptoms wax and wane relative to daily stress—we have been studying the function of stress response systems," she says.

Although we may feel we are in chaos when confronted with stress, our bodies have a well-defined set of "emergency procedures." The success of these procedures lies in hormones. Perhaps the most familiar result of stress hormones is the rush of adrenaline that we feel when frightened. Secreted by the adrenal glands, adrenaline pumps up heart and respiration rates, preparing us to run for our lives or stand and fight. Less dramatic—but equally essential to survival—are the hormones of the hypothalamic-pituitary-adrenal (HPA) axis—one of the main stress response axes that ensure that the mind can focus and the body can respond to stress. Dr. Crofford's team is exploring the difference between people who take stress in stride and those who will be throttled by a painful fibromyalgia attack.

Dr. Crofford's team has found that hormone secretion on the HPA axis occurs differently in people with fibromyalgia. Compared to others, people with fibromyalgia have increased pituitary hormone activity and blunted adrenal activity after the axis is stimulated. She and her co-workers have also found differences in the circadian rhythms, or schedule, on which hormones are secreted. Normally, hormone secretion is active in the early morning, tapers off during the day, is quiet in the evening, and is "turned on" for emergency response by stress. In people with fibromyalgia, however, this secretion schedule is altered. This may help to explain why people with fibromyalgia tend to have difficult mornings.

These stress-response systems are critical to the integration of the mind and body. Many of the symptoms of fibromyalgia—sleep disturbance, fatigue, difficulty concentrating—are tied to the brain and could influence or be influenced by stress hormones. Dr. Crofford also notes that stress can alter blood flow and muscle metabolism.

"It's not yet clear how all the findings of hormone and neurochemical disturbances fit together," says Dr. Crofford. She suspects many trails— her work with stress hormones, Dr. Bennett's work on growth hormones, and Dr. Russell's research on serotonin and substance P—may eventually meet on the way to finding a cause or causes for fibromyalgia.

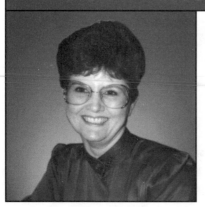

My Attitude, My Choice
by Lynne Green
Broadway, NC

When I was diagnosed with fibromyalgia five years ago, I was so relieved to be able to put a name on the miserable fatigue and chronic pain that had plagued my life for so long. Exercise, a good diet, and chiropractic care helped me lead a normal life without too much difficulty until last year when my flares became more frequent and severe.

Since my condition has worsened, I have had to work especially hard at keeping a positive attitude and remaining optimistic about my future. To do this, I've learned to adapt my lifestyle in a way that allows me to get the most out of life. I set short-term goals for myself so I am motivated to stay active. I know I must take frequent rest breaks, particularly when I have activities planned that require a lot of energy. Accepting limitations was difficult for me, but once I did, I became free to enjoy more fully the things I can do.

It is so important for those of us with fibromyalgia to keep a positive attitude. As far as we know, there is little we can control about the flares and all the other symptoms that occur, but we can still control how we think.

CHAPTER TWO

Treatments

Based on emerging research findings, people with fibromyalgia have reason for hope. Today's treatment regimen focuses first on restorative sleep—a goal that can be achieved for most with medications initially developed for depression—and gradual reconditioning of muscles through exercise.

Children with fibromyalgia will typically be treated in much the same manner as adults. However, the effectiveness of these treatments has yet to be proven in juveniles. The Arthritis Foundation is currently funding research to determine if adult treatment measures are optimal for juveniles, or if another approach will provide more lasting outcomes.

An Overview of Options

Although fibromyalgia has no known cure, its effects can be reduced. Mild symptoms may require minimum treatment and avoidance of what worsens them. But most people will benefit from a comprehensive care program, including:

- medications, to diminish pain and improve sleep
- exercise, to stretch muscles and improve cardiovascular fitness
- relaxation techniques, to ease tense muscles
- education, to help understand and cope with the condition
- healthy habits, such as eating well and giving up smoking.

Each of these techniques will be discussed in depth in individual chapters. The following general overview is an introduction to them, allowing you to determine which you'd like to learn more about and to compare treatments to your own current regimen.

Medications

Tricyclic Antidepressants

Traditionally used for treating depression, tricyclic antidepressants in smaller doses can also be effective in treating fibromyalgia. By relaxing muscles and promoting better sleep, they can help people with fibromyalgia break out of the chronic pain-fatigue symptom cycle.

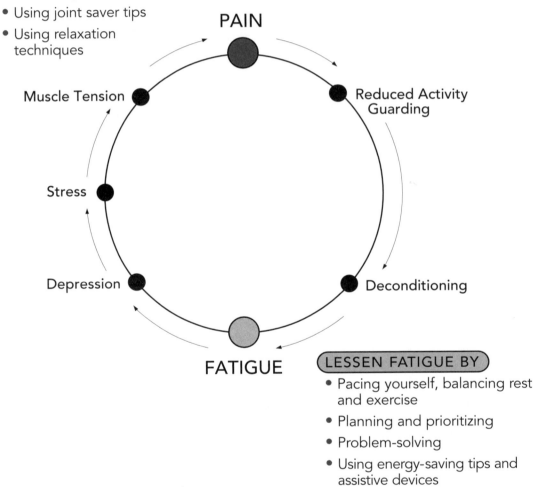

LESSEN PAIN BY

- Exercising
- Putting heat or cold on sore joints
- Taking your medications as your doctor says
- Using joint saver tips
- Using relaxation techniques

PAIN

Muscle Tension

Reduced Activity Guarding

Stress

Depression

Deconditioning

FATIGUE

LESSEN FATIGUE BY

- Pacing yourself, balancing rest and exercise
- Planning and prioritizing
- Problem-solving
- Using energy-saving tips and assistive devices

THE PAIN/FATIGUE CYCLE
Tricyclic antidepressants that relax muscles and promote sleep help people with fibromyalgia break out of the chronic pain—fatigue cycle.

Examples of tricyclic antidepressants include: amitriptyline *(Elavil)*, doxepin *(Sinequan)*, and nortriptyline *(Pamelor)*. Results vary greatly from person to person. Possible side effects include daytime drowsiness, constipation, dry mouth, and increased appetite and weight gain.

SSRIs (Selective Serotonin Re-uptake Inhibitors)

Newer antidepressants, used alone or in combination with tricyclic antidepressants to treat fibromyalgia, include fluoxetine *(Prozac)*, sertraline *(Zoloft)*, and paroxetine *(Paxil)*. The results of studies on their effectiveness are mixed—one group found them helpful, citing the drugs' beneficial effect on the uptake of serotonin. Researchers think that people with fibromyalgia are unable to properly metabolize serotonin, a hormone important for pain modulation and maintenance of the deep stage of sleep (see Serotonin in this chapter). However, another study found no benefit from these drugs for people with fibromyalgia. And they do have side effects, including insomnia in some people—an effect that could worsen fibromyalgia symptoms. Future studies on the drugs will provide definitive answers.

Nonsteroidal Anti-Inflammatory Drugs (NSAIDs)

This group of drugs, which includes aspirin, ibuprofen, and naproxen, relieves pain by fighting inflammation. Since inflammation is not a symptom of fibromyalgia, these medications don't have a major effect on the condition. However, moderate doses may help relieve pain and stiffness. NSAID side effects include stomach upset and peptic ulcers.

Acetaminophen and Noninflammation Analgesics

Acetaminophen

Acetaminophen, a noninflammation analgesic, is useful for those who wish to avoid aspirin and other NSAIDS. As with NSAIDs, acetaminophen bestows only a minor benefit against fibromyalgia pain and stiffness. This common, over-the-counter drug is not without side effects. It can damage the liver when taken over a long period with another liver-toxic agent, such as alcohol.

Another agent is tramadol hydrochloride *(Ultram)*, a centrally acting analgesic with a minimal potential for addiction in patients with a tendency to addiction. Potential side effects of *Ultram* include nervousness, anxiety, and sleep disorder.

Narcotics

These potent drugs interrupt pain signals traveling to the brain by imitating the body's own endorphins, which block pain signals naturally. Examples include propoxyphene hydrochloride *(Darvon)*, codeine, hydrocodone *(Vicodin)*, demerol, and morphine. However, their addictive nature renders them problematic in the treatment of fibromyalgia's long-term chronic pain.

Corticosteroids

Used to treat some forms of arthritis such as rheumatoid arthritis and lupus, corticosteroids (e.g. *cortisone, prednisone*) are powerful anti-inflammatory agents. However, inflammation is not a fibromyalgia symptom, so corticosteroids have little effectiveness in the treatment of it. They also carry a risk of side effects such as weight gain and mood swings. These drugs are not the same as the performance-enhancing anabolic steroid drugs athletes sometimes use, which should also be avoided in treating fibromyalgia.

Tranquilizers

These can help reduce painful muscle tension and assist with sleep, and generally, they have been found to be helpful in fibromyalgia. However, they can be addictive if used for long periods of time. Use of tranquilizers should be carefully monitored by your physician. These drugs act on the brain thalamus and hypothalamus and exert a calming effect. Generally, tranquilizers are not used in fibromyalgia. Occasionally a sedative like zolpidem tartrate (*Ambien*) may be prescribed if sleep is the major problem and other approaches to sleep management have not helped. Here again, sedatives are also not usually prescribed.

Tender-Point Injections

A local anesthetic directly injected into a tender point can provide relief that lasts for anywhere from hours to several months. These injections are initially painful, and generally are used only in cases of severe or persistent tender-point pain.

Topical Ointments

Some topical "deep-heating" rubs may modify the sensation of pain and may increase blood flow in the skin, soothing the painful muscle. Such creams contain methyl salicylate. Creams that contain capsaicin, however, may be used along with other medications to temporarily modify joint pain or nerve pain. Capsaicin decreases the ability of nerve endings in the skin to sense pain. However, because capsaicin products must be applied two to three times a day, and because the areas affected by fibromyalgia are so extensive, they are not a practical management tool for widespread pain.

Other Treatments

Acupuncture

Many fibromyalgia patients try acupuncture, a Chinese practice of puncturing the body with needles at specific points to cure disease or relieve pain. Relief seldom lasts more than 24 hours.

Exercise and Physical Therapy

Regular exercise can help anyone feel better, but people with fibromyalgia can reap enormous benefits. Toned, well-conditioned muscles can diminish the pain of fibromyalgia, and aerobic fitness can improve sleep.

People with fibromyalgia may be reluctant to exercise if they are tired and in pain. Low- or nonimpact aerobic exercises such as brisk walking, biking, swimming, or water aerobics are a few ways to start exercising without jarring painful joints. Regular workouts, with gradually increased frequency, will guarantee a better level of fitness. Gently stretching muscles and moving joints daily before and after aerobics will increase exercise endurance. Chapter 10 presents a more in-depth look at exercise and its benefits for people with fibromyalgia.

Doctors may also prescribe physical therapy, which can include a specific exercise program, as well as such pain-management techniques as heat, ice, massage, whirlpool, ultrasound, TENS and biofeedback.

Rest and Relaxation

In a hectic world, it's often difficult to take time out for rest. But it's important for people with fibromyalgia to do just that. Rest and relaxation (both physical and mental) allow the body time to heal itself, breaking the vicious cycle of pain, stress, and depression. Everyone, but particularly people with fibromyalgia, needs to balance periods of activity with periods of rest.

Education

People with fibromyalgia can be their own best researchers and advocates. By learning about the condition, and taking an active role in their care, they can lead healthy lives. Reading this book—and any other reliable material about fibromyalgia—is a good first step. Others include asking the doctor questions to ensure understanding and create a dialogue, as well as seeking out support groups and classes like the Fibromyalgia Self-Help Course, organized by the Arthritis Foundation, to boost knowledge and coping skills.

Healthy Habits

The first step toward becoming a healthy person may be to act like one. Pain and depression can lead some people with fibromyalgia to eat poorly, or seek relief in cigarettes or alcohol, which may actually worsen symptoms in the long run. Giving up such unhealthy habits as drinking too much and smoking can be the first step to an overall renewal, allowing the body to devote all its energy to recovering from fibromyalgia. And replacing a junky, fast-food diet with good-tasting, healthy food will not only help the person eating it feel better, but ensure that his body gets the fuel and vitamins it needs—without too much salt or fat—to battle fibromyalgia.

PART TWO
Taking Charge

This section, and the rest of the book, is about making the best use of what you've learned in Part One: how to take control of your life and health care. Along with the shift from education to action, you may notice another change: that the text addresses "you" instead of "a person with fibromyalgia." For the sake of direct communication, it's assumed that you, the reader, are the person with the condition— although family members are encouraged to read this book as well. Also, you'll hear from other voices, as everyday people contribute their experiences—and successes—with fibromyalgia.

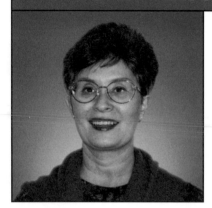

My Keys to Managing Fibromyalgia
by Arlene R. Gorski, RN
Herndon, VA

Learning to live with the complex, unpredictable symptoms of fibromyalgia syndrome has been an ongoing challenge for me. I was a nurse enjoying a multifaceted career before I was officially diagnosed several years ago, after years of elusive symptoms. Within a few months of diagnosis, I was forced to give up my livelihood as well as treasured relationships with friends and colleagues. I was unable to pursue hobbies I loved, and even my own body became a stranger to me. It was no simple matter to manage my illness while various professionals sought to "unlayer" my many symptoms.

To fight back, I began to learn everything I could about this mysterious, disabling illness. I sought out others with FMS (Fibromyalgia Syndrome) and became active with them in a self-help organization. Although these activities helped allay my fears, it was still difficult for me to rebuild my health or my life.

To my dismay, the very medical professionals who were treating me often had less information about the condition than I did. I realized it was imperative that I educate not only myself, but also the professionals who were treating me. I have personally done so in two ways: 1) by persistently sharing my knowledge and experience with my own medical treatment team, and 2) by networking with medical professionals through my fibromyalgia organization, other FMS groups, and related health organizations.

Despite my own frustrations, I have fought for mutual dialogue between patients and professionals to achieve a better understanding of a condition encased in dubious labels, misunderstandings, and ignorance. This is a cause that every fibromyalgia patient should adopt. Not only does commitment to fibromyalgia education lead to improved medical treatment and self-management, but it also provides broad rewards of personal growth, improved self-esteem, and strength in working with others toward a single goal: living a full life with fibromyalgia.

*Reprinted from **Arthritis Today**, January/February, 1995.*

CHAPTER THREE

Your Role as Self-Manager

When you're ill, it's sometimes easy to become passive, allowing others to make decisions and do things for you. With fibromyalgia, that could be a critical mistake. Therapy begins with action, first by learning about your condition, and then by doing something about it. It all begins when you take the reins at your "corporation"—which consists of your mind and body. Promote yourself to manager of your condition.

This chapter can help you sort out your priorities, with these main goals in mind:

- controlling your physical symptoms as much as possible
- meeting the emotional challenges of fibromyalgia
- living a full, independent life

Your Role as Parent of a Child with Fibromyalgia

If your child has fibromyalgia, it is crucial that family, friends, peers, and especially school officials understand the hidden aspects of the condition. You may want to talk with school officials about your child's condition and any functional difficulties that could be remedied with supplies or adaptive equipment.

For more information, contact your local chapter of the Arthritis Foundation to purchase a copy of *Educational Rights for Children with Arthritis-Related Conditions*. Studies so far are inconclusive on the effectiveness of adult medications on children with fibromyalgia, but it is important to encourage your child to remain active, get plenty of exercise and rest, and lead as normal a life as possible.

Five Habits of Successful Self-Managers

People who lead healthy lives with fibromyalgia have found innumerable, ingenious methods of dealing with the disorder, some of which you'll read about in this book. But these individuals all share a few distinctive traits. Here's how to emulate them:

1. Join Your Health-Care Team

If you don't have a doctor, get one immediately. (See "Finding a Physician" in Chapter 4.) Then become an active member of the team that's treating your fibromyalgia.

- Take part in planning your treatment program—and follow it. Remember that for fibromyalgia, treatment includes not only medication, but also (for most) exercise, stretching, and adequate rest.
- Write down questions, symptoms, problems, and concerns to ask your doctor so you don't forget them. Be brief and concise.
- Monitor your symptoms and report any changes to your doctor. For a full explanation of how to interact with your health-care team, see Chapter 4.

2. Assume Responsibility for What You Can Control

Synthesizing a healthy mind and body begins with taking responsibility for yourself. You are the only person who has control over your thoughts and actions. Leading a happy, healthy life with fibromyalgia requires committing yourself to doing everything you can to get better, even beyond a prescribed treatment program such as taking medication and exercising. Three basic skills can help you maintain independence:

- Set goals and work toward them (see "Goal Setting and Contracting" in this chapter).
- Get help when you need it. Try brainstorming with family and friends, or use the problem-solving techniques in this chapter. Ask questions, read a book, or seek professional guidance when you've exhausted your own methods of overcoming an obstacle.
- Accept what you can't control. Some problems and symptoms are not going to go away, and you'll have to find a way to come to terms with them.

3. *Learn as Much as You Can about Fibromyalgia*

- Keep informed about fibromyalgia by asking questions of your health-care team and reading as much reliable information about fibromyalgia as you can. This book is just one resource—check your local library and bookstores for others.
- Check with local hospitals, health maintenance organizations (HMOs), or other health-care facilities to find out what resources, such as classes and support groups, are available in your community.
- Check the Yellow Pages for the local office of the Arthritis Foundation (or call 800/283-7800) or your local fibromyalgia organization.
- See the Resources section of this book for additional information.

4. *Master Emotional Challenges*

- Practice stress-reduction and relaxation exercises. Besides promoting a pleasant, comfortable state of well-being, relaxation also helps your body balance itself by allowing a rest period in which it can heal.
- Talk over your feelings and problems with family and friends. Only by this kind of communication will they know first-hand what you're going through and be able to offer assistance or understanding.
- Educate your family and friends about the nature of fibromyalgia. Share interesting articles or books with them. If they have questions, suggest they accompany you to meet with your physician or another member of your health-care team.
- Seek outside help if your problems seem overwhelming. There are many sources of assistance in every community; keep asking until you find one that fits your needs.

5. *Develop a Wellness Lifestyle*

If you don't feel healthy, imitate the habits of a healthy person. You may find that the feeling rubs off.

- Exercise regularly and eat a balanced diet of good-tasting foods.
- Get plenty of rest.
- Do things that make you happy and your life richer.
- Adopt a positive attitude. (See Chapter 12.)

HABITS OF SUCCESSFUL SELF-MANAGERS

1. Join your health-care team.

2. Assume responsibility for what you can control.

3. Learn as much as you can about fibromyalgia.

4. Manage emotional challenges.

5. Develop a wellness lifestyle.

A Note on Grief and Depression

Mental and emotional health play strong roles in the battle against fibromyalgia, more so than in many other physical conditions. There is a link between the disorder and depression, with studies showing approximately one quarter of people with fibromyalgia are clinically depressed, requiring care under the supervision of a mental-health professional. No one knows if depression is a cause or effect of the disorder, but depression can be overcome. It's difficult to take command of your life and health care—a must if you are to get better—if you're already feeling overwhelmed and defeated.

If you've recently been diagnosed with fibromyalgia, you may be grieving the loss of the life you had before symptoms set in. That's natural when you're faced with a chronically painful condition for which there is no cure. Talking to friends and family may help. But if you find you're depressed and crying frequently for more than two weeks, see a doctor. Other signs that you may need professional help for depression include thoughts of hurting yourself or others, or persistent, unshakable feelings of worthlessness. See "Depression: A Self-Test" in Chapter 9.

If your depression isn't severe, you may be able to improve your emotional state by teaching that "little voice in your head" some new lines. Tips on breaking the habit of seeing things in black or white, of overgeneralizing, or of "catastrophizing" insignificant events are discussed in Chapter 9, where these subjects are covered in depth.

Don't allow negative thinking or depression to bar the way to getting better. Make sure the "head" of your corporation is a clear one, ready to take on the challenges of the future.

Goal Setting and Contracting

Like the manager of a business or organization, you must first know what you want to accomplish before charting a course of action. Goal setting can help you decide what's important in managing fibromyalgia.

Think of a goal as something you would like to accomplish in the next three to six months. Be realistic and very specific. Start by thinking of all the things you would like to do, then decide which of these things realistically can be done in the next several weeks or months. Remember, if you choose a goal too big or too far off, you may get discouraged and give up.

Goals usually need to be broken down into small, doable steps or tasks. For example, if your overall goal is to improve your physical fitness, smaller steps could include:

- making an appointment to see your doctor or physical therapist to get information on the types of exercise that would be best for your condition
- researching classes such as warm-water swimming classes or adaptive physical-education classes at the local Arthritis Foundation chapter, hospital, community college, or health club
- finding a friend to exercise with.

The next step is to get started. Decide which steps to work on and exactly when to do them.

ACTIVITY: Contracting for a Better Life with Fibromyalgia

To help map out a schedule for accomplishing your goals, you might try drawing up a weekly contract with yourself. Here are some key parts of such a contract:

- specific steps toward your overall goal
- specific plans about what you will do to fulfill your plan. For instance: What will you do? (List a specific behavior/activity; for example, walking); How much? (e.g., 15 minutes); When? (time of day, before or after meals, etc.); How often? (times per week).

For example, "Three times this week I will walk around the block before lunch."

Start slowly. In contracting, it's best to work on something you can do in one week. Don't begin by contracting to do things every day—three to four times a week is more realistic.

Using a scale of zero to ten, you should have a confidence level of seven or more that you will complete the entire contract. (Zero is totally unsure and ten is totally confident.)

Make copies of the Contract Form below to keep a record of your weekly goals.

To keep you motivated, have someone else—a family member, a friend, or perhaps a member of your health-care team—sign your contract.

CONTRACT FORM

THIS WEEK I WILL: **WEEK OF:**_____

FOR EXAMPLE: *This week I will walk around the block before lunch three times.*
　　　　　　　　　(WHAT)　(HOW MUCH)　(WHEN)　(HOW MANY)

WHAT
_____

HOW MUCH
_____

WHEN
_____

HOW MANY DAYS
_____

HOW CERTAIN ARE YOU

(On a scale of 0 to 10 with 0 being totally unsure and 10 being totally confident)

SIGNATURE:

Problem Solving

Problem-solving skills are essential to meeting your goals and setting realistic contracts. Try the Problem-Solving Work Sheet on page 31 if you're having trouble overcoming obstacles.

ACTIVITY: Using a Problem-Solving Work Sheet

1. Identify a problem fibromyalgia has caused in your life. What are the concerns? What caused them? Can they be broken down into smaller, more manageable issues? For example: "I used to have a lot of friends at work, but because of fibromyalgia, I've lost some of them. Early mornings are bad. I never feel well until I'm at the office for a couple of hours. It's worst when I'm responsible for the car pool—I have to get up earlier than ever, and then I feel worse."

2. List ideas to solve the problem. What do you want to achieve, and what can you do about it? Write down as many options as you can. Ask for suggestions from family, friends, and members of your health-care team, or community resources (consider them "freelance consultants" for your "corporation." For example: "I could apologize for my crankiness. I could take a hot bath for stiffness. Or dress more warmly. I could check with my doctor on new medications. I could drop out of the car pool. Or quit my job. Or I could check with my supervisor to see if I could work out a 'flex-time' schedule, beginning and ending my day a bit later."

3. Consider the pros and cons. What are the consequences of each option? What are the advantages and disadvantages? Rank their order from least to most practical and desirable. Example: "I should and will apologize for my crankiness. But that won't make mornings easier. Taking a hot bath would mean getting up even earlier—ugh. Dressing more warmly doesn't always work. The doctor recently gave me a new medication, and I want to give it a fair trial before switching it. Dropping out of the car pool means no longer afflicting my coworkers with my ill humor, but doesn't solve the problem. I can't quit—I need my job, and more importantly, it allows me to remain independent. My supervisor might be open to having me come in later and stay later—she's often had trouble finding people to finish up a few last-minute items."

4. Select one option and develop a plan to implement it. Example: "I'll ask my supervisor about it. She's usually most receptive to

new ideas right around the mid-morning coffee break. Hmmm, perhaps I'll take in some coffee cake tomorrow. Maybe that will help melt the chill from my former friends, too."

5. Do it! Put your plan into action. Remember that change can be difficult. Be sure to give your idea a fair chance before deciding it won't work.

6. Evaluate the results. After you have given your idea a fair chance, look at the results. Has your problem been solved? Are you headed in the right direction in working toward your goal? If not, choose another idea from your list and try again. Example: "After I switched to a flex-time schedule, there were a couple of trade-offs I hadn't foreseen. It's usually too late to go out after work, and I have to miss the evening news. Sometimes I'm so tired when I get home I'm out with the lights. But overall, it's been well worth it. Now my body has a couple of hours to loosen up before work, and I almost feel like a human being when I get there. Not surprisingly, I'm getting along with everyone—including my husband—much better."

7. Accept that the problem may not be solvable immediately. If none of your ideas works now, try them again later. Most importantly, don't feel discouraged. Keep going and look for alternate paths to what you want to accomplish.

PROBLEM—SOLVING WORK SHEET

1. Select a current problem or concern and list any known causes.
2. Write down several possible solutions for dealing with this problem or its causes.
3. Consider the advantages and disadvantages of each option.
4. Select an option to try.
5. Evaluate your results after implementing the option selected.

① PROBLEM/CAUSE:

② POSSIBLE SOLUTIONS   **③ ADVANTAGES**   **DISADVANTAGES**

④ OPTION TO TRY   **⑤ RESULTS/OUTCOME**

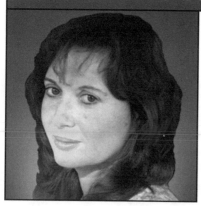

The Write Solution
by Evelyn Schuman
Merlin, OR

I've experienced many lifestyle changes due to fibromyalgia syndrome. But during the process of reinventing my life, I discovered the joy of writing. Writing has provided a creative outlet to vent conflicting emotions—a private place to sound off and regain my equilibrium. I can explore feelings and gather scattered thoughts, putting my world back into perspective. Writing serves as an escape hatch from the daily restrictions of life with fibromyalgia. I can transcend the prison of pain while writing a poem, or laugh at a limerick dancing in my head.

Life with a chronic illness can isolate you and drive a wedge through your relationships. As a solution, I rely on the therapeutic value of expressing myself through a personal essay. It has strengthened communication with friends and family when spoken words were inadequate. Putting down negative emotions on paper releases bottled-up anger, and dissolves any destructive self-pity.

Although I'm not currently competing for the next Pulitzer prize, writing gives me the thrill of accomplishment without much physical effort. During a relapse, when my motto for the day is "I'm up and I'm dressed, what else do you want?," I can still jot down a few lines and boost my sagging spirits.

The diversion of creative writing has brought a touch of excitement and fun to some fairly mundane days. My journal has become a confidante who doesn't get annoyed when I whine about pain or fatigue. And most of all, there's no hefty psychotherapy bill to pay at the end of the month!

Recording Your Experiences

Why Should I Keep a Journal?

In *Opening Up: The Healing Power of Confiding in Others,* James Pennebaker showed that people with chronic illness who wrote about their painful feelings and losses in some type of journal reported fewer symptoms, fewer visits to the doctor, fewer days off work, improved mood and outlook, and even enhanced immune function.

Keeping records of your experiences with fibromyalgia can make a difference in your health. Many people find it useful to write them in a journal or diary, along with other observations. You may also find it helpful to share them with your physician or health-care provider. A written record of your experiences, whether a journal, diary, or self-monitoring work sheet, can benefit you in these ways:

- provide you with concrete documentation of your subjective symptoms
- help you in communicating with your doctors
- help you with explanations to family, friends, coworkers, or employers
- help you understand your disease more fully and identify your symptom patterns throughout the year
- help you identify factors that trigger symptoms and fluctuations
- provide you with a good, more objective memory aid
- help you "process" your symptoms, feelings, and thoughts and let them go, freeing your mind to focus on healing
- provide a faithful friend and ready listener
- help you reassert control.

ACTIVITY: Keeping a Journal

On the following pages, we'll provide different methods for you to experiment with for recording your symptoms and experiences with fibromyalgia. You may want to try keeping a *Symptoms Diary* and/or a *Thoughts Diary.* You may choose to keep records of your exercise activities in the *Exercise Diary.* A weekly *Time Analysis Work Sheet* is provided to help you analyze how you spend a typical week. Try different techniques until you find one that's practical and easy to use.

Here are some guidelines for writing and recording your symptoms and experiences: Monitor only what is important to you—not what you think you ought to care about. Below are some factors to consider:

- amount/location of pain
- level of energy/fatigue
- hours of sleep/rest
- medications and their side effects
- unusual symptoms
- stress/problems
- exercise
- activity level
- food intake
- weight
- positive experiences
- mood changes
- thoughts/reactions to daily events
- something funny you saw or heard that day.

Keeping a journal, like any new habit, will take a while to feel natural. To give it a fair trial, set a schedule, such as five to 10 minutes, three times a week. If you like it, you'll probably find yourself writing on a regular basis. Select a method that fits your schedule and needs. Here are a few strategies:

- Record a running symptom log in a calendar, diary, or notebook. Enter symptoms daily or weekly as needed during flares or times of uncertainty.
- Write (or use a typewriter, computer, or tape recorder if writing is too painful) about your experiences with fibromyalgia and your reactions to these experiences. One woman simply started writing down all her disease symptoms along with her deepest feelings and thoughts about her condition.
- Divide a sheet of paper in half and record all of the "facts" of the day—problems, challenges, or positive experiences—on one side. On the other side, record your emotional reactions and thoughts about these events. Logs like these are very useful for emotional release as well as for self-discovery.
- Select only a few symptoms to monitor initially, such as your pain level, fatigue level, and mood. Use a Symptoms Diary to keep track of changes. A tool that shows how symptoms change over time can help you see the interrelationships among these symptoms.

- Date your entries so that you can look back over them and see patterns and progress.
- Write freely and selfishly. Don't worry about grammar or misspellings. Keep this diary to yourself—you'll write more honestly.
- Write to develop insight into your feelings—it can be an emotional release. But don't write to avoid taking needed action.

SAMPLE THOUGHTS DIARY

DATE/TIME	UNPLEASANT EMOTION	SITUATION	SELF-TALK	RATIONAL RESPONSE
AUGUST 3 9:30 a.m.	depressed, frustrated	In kitchen looking at mess.	I'll never get this kitchen clean.	I'll just do a little bit and get started. There's no reason I have to do it all today.
AUGUST 4 10:15 a.m.	tired, discouraged	Putting dishes away.	I should have done a better job of straightening up.	Nothing in the world is perfect, but I did make the room look better.
AUGUST 6 1:00 p.m.	frustrated	Phone rings and wakes me up from nap.	I should have taken the phone off the hook. I never do anything right.	Nonsense! I do lots of things right. Most days I remember to take the phone off the hook.
AUGUST 7 3:00 p.m.	depressed	Expected call from friend - it didn't come.	I have no real friends. She should have called by now.	My friends are just as real as anyone's. Who says she "should" have called me. I think I'll call her.

THOUGHTS DIARY

To appreciate the power of your self-talk and the part it plays in your emotional life, make your own thoughts diary. Make a notation each time you experience an unpleasant emotion. Include everything you tell yourself to keep the emotion going.

DATE/TIME	UNPLEASANT EMOTION	SITUATION	SELF-TALK	RATIONAL RESPONSE

SYMPTOMS DIARY

It is useful to monitor your pain level and mood to learn more about possible associations. Use the chart below to rate your current mood and pain level on the 0-10 scale. For the next week, rate your pain and mood three times per day (e.g. AM — when you get up in the morning, Midday, and PM — before going to bed), then look for patterns or possible associations.

FOR EACH TIME PERIOD
- Mark an X across from the number that describes your mood; (0=best mood, 10=worst mood or most anxious/depressed/negative feelings).
- Mark an 0 across from the rating of pain; (0=no pain, 10=worst pain).

MOOD/PAIN DIARY

	AM	Mid-Day	PM	AM	Mid-Day	PM	AM	Mid-Day	PM	AM	Mid-Day	PM	AM	Mid-Day	PM	AM	Mid-Day	PM	AM	Mid-Day	PM
10																					
9																					
8																					
7																					
6																					
5																					
4																					
3																					
2																					
1																					
0																					
	Monday/Day 1			Tuesday/Day 2			Wednesday/Day 3			Thursday/Day 4			Friday/Day 5			Saturday/Day 6			Sunday/Day 7		

EXERCISE DIARY

Use this chart to keep records of your exercise activities.

DATE/TIME	EXERCISES	FREQUENCY/ DURATION	PERCEIVED EXERTION OR HEART RATE	FEELINGS/ COMMENTS

WEEKLY TIME ANALYSIS WORK SHEET

Use the following work sheet to help you analyze how you spend a typical week.

	Monday	Tuesday	Wednesday	Thursday	Friday	Saturday	Sunday
6 a.m.							
7 a.m.							
8 a.m.							
9 a.m.							
10 a.m.							
11 a.m.							
noon							
1 p.m.							
2 p.m.							
3 p.m.							
4 p.m.							
5 p.m.							
6 p.m.							
7 a.m.							
9 p.m.							
8 p.m.							
9 p.m.							
10 p.m.							
11 p.m.							
midnight							

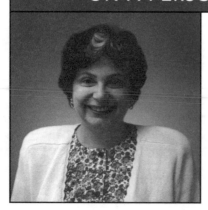

Don't Dawdle!
By Jane A. Zanca
Decatur, GA

First, I saw my internist. He sent me to a rheumatologist, someone he "knew." It was three months before "Dr. Dawdle" could see me. The wait in Dr. Dawdle's lobby was two and a half hours. No kidding. You can imagine how painful that was.

Inside, at last, Dr. Dawdle interrupted my narrative, dismissed a loudly crackling shoulder, and jabbed a trigger point. Pain shot through me. "Yep," he said, "fibromyalgia." He scribbled prescriptions and whisked out. Ten minutes. That's it.

I told my internist. "But Dr. Dawdle is a nice guy!" he exclaimed. "Doctors who are good with doctors are not necessarily good with patients," I said. "Please refer me to someone else." Within three weeks, "Dr. Betsy" saw me — promptly.

She reviewed my entire health history, asked if I had experienced depression, made careful notes, and examined my joints as well as my muscles. Before touching a trigger point, she warned, "This may hurt." Then she explained her findings, the lab work I needed, and my medications. She gave me a brochure on fibromyalgia and asked if I had any questions. We shared a laugh because we were both having a bad hair day.

Thirty minutes. That's everything. If you ask me about a good rheumatologist, which one do you think I'll recommend? Don't Dawdle. Get a good doctor now. It makes all the difference in the world.

CHAPTER FOUR

Dealing with Your Doctor

Finding a Physician

If you don't have a doctor, find one immediately. If you know people with fibromyalgia who are happy with their treatment, ask them for their doctors' names. Or contact the local Arthritis Foundation for advice. The Foundation can also supply an arthritis specialists referral list. But don't simply call the first name on the list. Interview a few doctors to determine their knowledge of, interest in, and attitude toward fibromyalgia. (See "Searching for a Top Doc?" in this chapter.)

Remember that you're looking for a partner to join your health-care team. A good partnership depends on trusting your doctor's knowledge and abilities—and on liking him or her. To discover which qualities are most important to you, think about the doctors you have visited in the past. What did you like or dislike about them? What qualities would the "ideal" doctor possess?

Your doctor will guide you in managing the physical aspects of living with fibromyalgia, most likely recommending:

- a balance of rest and activity
- an exercise program
- medications
- as needed, referral to a rheumatologist (a doctor who specializes in treating people with fibromyalgia and rheumatic diseases) or other medical specialists, depending on your symptoms, or to a physical or occupational therapist, nurse/patient educator, or counselor.

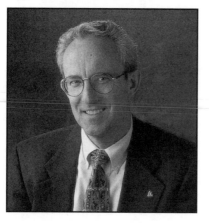

by Doyt L. Conn, MD

During his 25 years at the Mayo Clinic in Rochester, Minnesota, Doyt L. Conn, MD, was considered one of the country's top doctors in treating arthritis. As the Arthritis Foundation's senior vice president for medical affairs, Dr. Conn is also the chief medical authority for **Arthritis Today**. *Long acknowledged to be a leader in the fields of both arthritis research and patient care, Dr. Conn shares his own views on choosing a good doctor.*

The saying "You can't judge a book by its cover" is good advice for dealing with just about anybody. Now I'd like to suggest my own adage that applies to one important relationship: "You can't judge a doctor by a book."

Numerous books and magazines have published listings of doctors considered to be the best in their fields. In fact, we considered printing in **Arthritis Today** an excerpt from a book that listed rheumatologists and orthopedic surgeons considered by their peers to be top doctors. Then we decided against it.

I don't believe that books are the way to select a doctor. Yes, they do provide at least one bit of valuable information—the doctor's specialty. But that may be where their value ends. The problem with these books arises, in part, from the way the lists are generated. Many create their lists by surveying medical school department chairmen about who they consider to be the top doctors of their medical centers.

Often those recommendations are based on the papers the doctor publishes, the research he performs and the presentations he makes at scientific meetings. Unfortunately, they may have very little to do with the doctor's most important role—treating patients.

So how can you tell who will best perform this important role? My own experience in working with patients and with other doctors has led me to a few additional—and admittedly more subjective—criteria.

First, as a doctor who benefitted immeasurably from interaction with colleagues, medical students, and residents as well as with a diverse group of patients, I am convinced such interactions enhance a doctor's ability. Although a university medical center, in many ways, is probably the best location for a doctor to have this interaction, a large medical practice runs a close second. For a doctor in a solo practice, such opportunities are limited.

Experience is also critical in the making of a good doctor. Some people would argue that a young doctor fresh out of medical residency could provide you with the best, state-of-the-art treatment, but I believe an experienced doctor who keeps up with current knowledge is best, particularly for a patient with a chronic disease. Though my own training was important and prepared me well to begin medical practice, I believe that I became a better doctor over the years.

Perhaps even more important than a doctor's years of experience is where his experience lies. Many doctors at universities spend a great deal of time conducting research, publishing studies, and overseeing students' and residents' training. All of these activities keep the doctor current in his knowledge—a definite plus—but, unfortunately, they often preclude a lot of patient contact. Many doctors in research hospitals spend no more than one day a week seeing patients, which might be OK for a doctor who has already had many years of one-on-one experience with patients. I would not recommend selecting a doctor who spends more time doing research than seeing patients, particularly if the doctor has not been practicing very long.

And finally, there is one more quality of a top doctor that can't be conveyed in any book. It's often referred to as bedside manner and encompasses the doctor's willingness and ability to listen to your concerns, fears, and questions, and respond appropriately. It includes his willingness to let you take part in your treatment decisions. It is his concern for you and his ability to convey this concern while providing you the best possible care that matters the most.

Like the other qualities I have mentioned, bedside manner doesn't stand alone. There are plenty of unscrupulous but charismatic people out there promoting useless health-care products and procedures. But if you can separate those people from medically-trained professionals who have spent years dedicated to patient care, I am confident that you can find a top doc.

*Originally appeared in **Arthritis Today,** July/August 1996.*

Help Your Health-Care Team, Help Yourself!

Managing your fibromyalgia also means taking an active role with your doctor and other health-care professionals. Communication needs to be two-way to help ensure the best fit between your doctor's recommendations for treatment and your own goals and preferences. The relationship with your doctor is, in some respects, like a marriage partnership—allow plenty of room for give and take, and expect disagreements as well as agreements. Both parties need to work at it and show respect for each other for the relationship to succeed.

Who Makes Up Your Health-Care Team?

Many health professionals may be involved in your care, depending on your condition and their availability in your area. Following is a list of health-care professionals who may play a role in your treatment.

Doctors

Family physicians, general practitioners, and **primary-care physicians** provide medical care for adults and children with different types of arthritis and related conditions. These doctors also can help you find a specialist, if necessary.

Internists specialize in internal medicine and in treating adult diseases. They provide general care to adults and often help select specialists. Internists should not be confused with interns, who are doctors doing a year's training in a hospital after graduating from medical school.

Rheumatologists specialize in treating people with arthritis or related diseases that affect the joints, muscles, bones, skin, and other tissues. You may be referred to a rheumatologist if you need special care or treatment. Most rheumatologists are internists who have had further training in the care of people with arthritis and related diseases. Some rheumatologists also have pediatrics training.

Pediatricians treat childhood diseases. **Physiatrists** (fiz-eye-a-trists) may direct your physical therapy and rehabilitation. **Psychiatrists** (sy-ky-a-trists) are medical doctors who treat mental or emotional problems that need special attention. They can prescribe medications for treating the problems, as opposed to **psychologists** (see Other Health Professionals), who are also trained to treat mental or emotional problems, but have a doctor of philosophy rather (PhD) than a medical degree (MD) and therefore cannot prescibe medications.

Other Health Professionals

Some **nurses** are trained in arthritis and related illnesses and can assist your doctor with your treatment. They also help teach you about your treatment program and can answer many of your questions.

Occupational therapists can teach you how to reduce strain on your joints while doing everyday activities. They can fit you with splints and other devices to help reduce stress on your joints.

Pharmacists fill your prescriptions for medicines and can explain drugs' actions and side effects. Pharmacists can tell you how different medicines work together and answer questions about over-the-counter medicines.

Physical therapists can show you exercises to help keep your muscles strong and your joints from becoming stiff. They can help you learn how to use special equipment to move better. Some physical therapists also are trained to design individualized fitness programs for cardiovascular health maintenance and weight control.

Physicians assistants are trained, certified, and licensed to assist physicians by performing history taking, physical examination, diagnosis, and treatment of commonly encountered medical problems under the supervision of a licensed physician.

Podiatrists are specialists in foot care.

Psychologists can help you solve emotional or mental problems. Unlike psychiatrists, they do not have a medical degree and therefore cannot prescribe medication. They often work in conjunction with a physician or psychiatrist.

Social workers can help you find solutions to social and financial problems related to your disease.

"TAKE PART"

To get the most out of your contacts with your health-care team, remember to "Take PART":

P repare a list of questions, concerns, symptoms.

A sk questions.

R epeat what you have heard.

T ake action to reduce barriers to treatments.

Before Your Visit: Prepare

Following are some other steps to take before your visit:

- Make the appointment.
- Arrange to have your medical records transferred to the doctor's office if you are a new patient.
- Write down everything you want to ask or tell your doctor. Consider keeping a diary or journal. A "month-at-a-glance" calendar is a good way to keep a diary. Write out your questions in order of priority, realizing that probably only two or three may get answered during the visit. Time may not allow you to discuss everything, so highlight your most pressing concerns.
- Be prepared to describe the sequence and time when your symptoms usually begin to bother you. Use a self-monitoring form or a diary or other record sheet to keep track of your fibromyalgia symptoms between visits. Typical questions your doctor will ask include: Where are your symptoms? When did they start? Have they changed over time? How long have they lasted?
- Prepare a summary of what has happened since your last visit to the doctor. Your doctor might ask: Have you been following your treatment plan? How have you been feeling? Have you had any problems? What has been happening in your life? Jot down answers to these kinds of questions ahead of time.
- When evaluating a treatment, be sure you give it a fair trial before deciding it's a failure. It usually takes several weeks for a treatment to have a noticeable effect. Tell your doctor if you have trouble following recommendations.
- If, once you've given a treatment a fair trial, you don't seem to be getting better, tell your doctor or health team. Finding the right treatment often involves trial and error.
- Know the names and the dosages of all medicines you're taking, including prescription and over-the-counter drugs. If you're taking several medications, bring your pill bottles. This is especially important if you're visiting more than one doctor. If you are seeing your doctor on a return visit, make a list of any medication refills you need. Be prepared to discuss any medicines that are not helping or are causing side effects.

During the Visit: Ask, Repeat, and Take Action

Handle your doctor's visit like a business appointment. Come prepared, ask for what you need, repeat what you heard, and take action to deal with any barriers that may affect your treatment plan.

- Give your doctor a copy of your question list at the beginning of your appointment. Cover your most important concerns first, and be concise. Report to the doctor the reason for your visit and what you want him or her to do today.

- Tell the doctor about your symptoms, as well as changes in your life that may affect your fibromyalgia, your self-help activities, problems with treatment, results of visits to other health professionals, your current medications list, and any other updates that are relevant to your treatment plan. Be honest and give accurate information about your concerns, any unproven or alternative remedies you've tried, or changes you have made in your treatment regimen. Your doctor can safely recommend treatments only if he or she has the full picture.

- During the appointment, try to obtain any of the following information you do not already have:
  – your diagnosis and how your condition affects you
  – the purpose, risks and results of any tests
  – the choices for treatment and the benefits, risks, and side effects of each treatment option
  – when to call the doctor about side effects of your conditions or lack of response to a treatment
  – how a particular treatment should be performed.

- It's easy to forget or misunderstand instructions. Try repeating back to the physician the key points you've heard during the visit, like diagnosis, prognosis, next steps, treatment actions, and so on. This will allow your doctor to clarify anything that has been confusing and will help you remember what was discussed.

- Take notes or ask if the doctor has any written handouts or can give you written instructions about any prescribed treatments.

- Take part in decisions about treatment by sharing your goals and preferences. If there are barriers (financial concerns, conflicts with sleep or eating habits or daily schedule, and so on) to following your doctor's recommendations, let the doctor know.

- Remember that there is no single best treatment for everyone with fibromyalgia. Therefore, you must keep an open mind and work with your doctor. If something does not work, let your doctor know so together you can try something else. It may take a long time to find the right treatment.

ACTIVITY: Preparing for Your Doctor's Appointment

Use the following work sheets to prepare for your next appointment. Make copies if you need to so that you'll have them for future visits or for visits with other members of your health-care team. These can be guidelines to becoming an active participant in the treatment of your fibromyalgia.

"ASK THE DOCTOR" WORK SHEET

COMPLETE THIS PART **BEFORE** THE VISIT.

1. What is the main reason I am going to the doctor?
   _____
   _____

2. Is there anything else that concerns me about my health or treatment (e.g., effect of fibromyalgia on work, family, or mood; problems following the recommended treatment plan)?
   _____Yes_____No
   _____

3. What do I want the doctor to do today?
   _____
   _____

4. The symptoms that bother me the most are ... (What? Where? When did they start? Do they change over time? How long do they last?). NOTE: bring copies of any completed self-monitor ing forms/diaries.
   _____
   _____

5. What medications (prescriptions and over-the-counter) am I taking regularly? (List name(s) and dosage below or take the bottles to your appointment.)
   _____
   _____

6. What are my goals for treatment (what I want or expect to get out of treatment?)
   _____
   _____

7. Prepare and prioritize a list of questions to give the doctor early in the visit.
   _____
   _____
   _____

8. Do I need Medicare, Medicaid or other insurance cards/forms today?   _____Yes _____ No
   _____

"ASK THE DOCTOR" WORK SHEET

QUESTIONS TO ASK YOUR DOCTOR **DURING** THE VISIT.

1. What is happening to me? How is my fibromyalgia likely to affect me?
   _____
   _____

2. What are the results of my tests and what do they mean? May I have a copy of the results?
   _____

3. Why do I need the lab tests or X-rays that you are recommending today?
   _____

4. Are there any risks from these tests?
   _____

5. When should I call for the results?
   _____

6. What should I do at home (diet, activity, treatment options, special instructions, medications, precautions, etc.)?
   _____
   _____

   a. What are the benefits, costs and drawbacks (or risks) for each option for treatment?
      _____

   b. How and how often do I do the treatment?
      _____

   c. How long should I give it a try?
      _____

7. When should I call if my condition doesn't get better and the treatment does not seem to be working? What additional symptoms would warrant my calling before my next scheduled visit?
   _____
   _____

8. When should I return for another visit?
   _____

"ASK THE DOCTOR" WORK SHEET

MEDICATION QUESTIONS:

1. What is the name of the drug?_____

2. What are the purpose and benefits of this drug?
   _____

3. How quickly does it work? How long should I take this drug?
   _____

4. What are the possible side effects or drawbacks to the drug?
   _____

   a. When should I contact you about side effects?
      _____

   b. What can I do to prevent or deal with the side effects or drawbacks?
      _____

5. Is it all right to take the drug with other drugs (such as cold, sinus, allergy, pain medicines) I am taking?
   _____Yes_____No _____

6. When is the best time to take the drug? Before, with or after meals?_____

7. What should I do if I forget to take my medicine?
   _____

8. Are there any changes I should make in my diet?_____Yes_____No
   If so, what?_____

   a. Can I drink alcohol while taking this drug? _____Yes_____No_____

   b. Are there any other restrictions? _____Yes_____No
      If so, what?_____

8. Should I avoid driving or any other activity while taking this drug? _____Yes_____No
   _____

10. Is a generic drug available? If so, is the generic form as effective? _____Yes_____No
    _____

PART THREE

Helping Yourself

This section provides self help for the most common symptoms and emotional side effects of fibromyalgia.

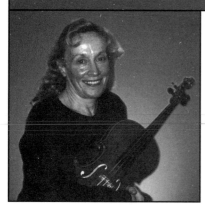

Just Keep on Playing
by Peggy LaVake
Cedar Grove, N.J.

I live with lupus and fibromyalgia and have many days when I ask myself, "How can I live the rest of my life feeling this way?" On those days, I feel alone and hopeless and wonder how I will handle the future with a silent disability.

Recently, I planned to host a small gathering of musician friends at my new apartment. It would be an evening of music-making—something I love to do. The day of the party I awoke feeling unrested, sore, and stiff as I almost always do. I knew I had a busy evening ahead of me, so I carefully structured my day in order to feel as good as possible. I made sure I was rested, knowing I would need every ounce of strength I could muster for the evening to be a success in my eyes.

When the guests arrived, we settled in to play. A chill of apprehension went down my spine as I realized I was already feeling tired and in pain, but still had two hours of playing and socializing ahead of me. I pushed the negative thoughts out of my head and played on. The more I played, the more I became absorbed in every note and nuance, and my fear quickly fell away.

Before I knew it our music-making session was over, and we gathered at the kitchen table for refreshments. All the while, I felt as if I had stumbled upon an answer to a question I constantly ask myself: "How do you live with a silent disability?" For me, the answer is simply to stay in the moment and keep on playing.

It doesn't have to be playing music—it can be any activity. When we are engaged in doing something we enjoy, our illness seems to fall away, if only for a short period of time. We can experience joyous moments and freedom from pain.

It's such a simple solution, but so hard to live by. We can't wait around until we feel better to start living our lives. Instead, we must live to the fullest despite how we feel.

Reprinted from *Arthritis Today*, March/April 1995.

CHAPTER FIVE

Managing Pain

For most people with fibromyalgia, medication for pain is limited to aspirin, other over-the-counter NSAIDs, or acetaminophen, with minor results. The most effective prescriptions are usually antidepressants that promote sleep, thus breaking the vicious pain-fatigue cycle. Addictive, narcotic painkillers are of little use in the long-term treatment of a chronic condition like fibromyalgia. For a full explanation of medications, see Chapter 2.

There are measures besides your doctor's prescriptions that can lessen pain. And there are measures that can worsen it—emotional reactions like stress can trigger a downward spiral of diminishing health. The following chapters offer ways you can break the pain-fatigue cycle. Following this chapter on pain, you'll find advice on how to deal with fatigue, get a better night's sleep, and manage stress.

What Is Pain?

Pain is your body's alarm system, signaling you when something is wrong. When part of your body is injured or damaged, nerves in that area release chemical signals. The nerves act like tiny telephone wires and send these signals to your brain, where they are recognized as pain. This process stimulates the formation and release of endorphins (naturally occurring painkilling substances).

Pain "tells" you that you need to do something. It generally either tells you to do it in a hurry (as in the acute pain you feel when you touch a hot stove) to prevent further injury, or sends a stubborn, but lower-key general distress signal (as in fibromyalgia's chronic pain). Chronic pain may be telling you something's wrong, but interpreting the pain is usually more difficult. If the chronic pain is due to fibromyalgia, your body may be telling you it needs rest, medications, relaxation, exercise, and possibly other strategies.

As a wise person once said, "Pain may be inevitable, but misery is optional." There is no magic solution to get rid of chronic pain, but you can manage it. It helps if you think of your pain as a signal for action, rather than an ordeal to be endured.

The Gate Theory of Pain

Pain can illogically vanish—people with severe injuries may initially feel nothing. Or it can flare without apparent reason, traveling unpredictably to uninjured parts of the body. The Gate Theory is an attempt to explain why this happens. It proposes that as pain signals travel to the brain, they pass a "pain gate" that can be opened or closed by various factors.

Factors that can "close" the gate and block pain signals include nerve impulses and endorphins. Certain medicines, such as morphine and other narcotic pain relievers, imitate the body's endorphins and block the pain signal. Techniques that block your perception of pain include stimulation of the skin in or near the area of pain with heat or cold, acupuncture, liniment, or electrical stimulation such as biofeedback. Similarly, positive stimuli, such as pleasant thoughts and humor, can alleviate pain by distracting from it.

On the other hand, negative emotional experiences, such as stress, mental and physical fatigue, anxiety, and depression can "open" the gate and intensify the perception of pain. That's why your pain can seem worse if you feel depressed, tired, or stressed.

Pain Gate "Openers"

Painful Habits

It's easy to slip into the habit of taking more medicines or drinking alcohol to escape pain. But ironically, these may actually worsen your symptoms by degrading your general health or deepening anxieties, depression, and fatigue. If you answer "yes" to any of the questions below, you may need to find new ways to handle pain.

- Do you use up pain medication faster than you used to?
- Do you drink alcohol several times a day?
- Do you spend all day in bed?
- Do you talk about pain or fibromyalgia much of the time?
- Do you smoke to relax?
- Do you feel as though your life is just one big chore?

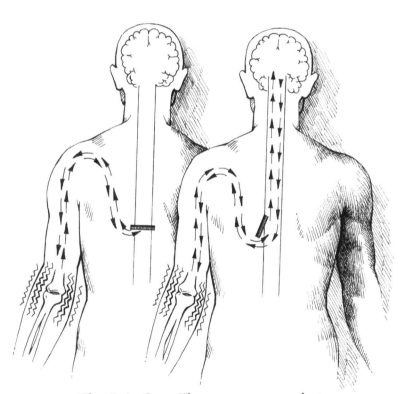

The Pain Gate Theory proposes that as pain signals travel to the brain, they pass a "pain gate" that can be closed or opened by various factors.

WHAT CAN CLOSE THE GATE
(i.e., block pain signals)?

- heat or cold treatments
- positive attitude and pleasant thoughts
- exercise
- relaxation
- some medicines
- massage
- distraction
- pleasing sights
- acupuncture
- topical lotions
- electrical stimulation
- humor

WHAT CAN OPEN THE GATE
(i.e., make your pain feel worse)?

- stress
- dwelling on pain
- fatigue
- anxiety
- depression

Changing your "painful habits" will help you feel better. Try replacing an old, painful habit with a new, positive one. Then reward yourself. Discuss these habits with your doctor, nurse, or other health-care workers who specialize in pain management. They can also help you with strategies to stop smoking or cut down on alcohol.

A Note on Unproven Remedies

Unproven remedies are treatments that have not been scientifically tested for safety or effectiveness. Some of these remedies are health frauds that have no scientific basis for their claims. Others are new treatments that are still under study. They are considered unproven or experimental until repeated, controlled studies show they work and won't cause dangerous side effects. Examples of unproven remedies include copper bracelets, bee venom, black pearl and yucca.

People with chronic pain are prime targets for unproven remedies, because they always hope a new treatment will be discovered. Some unproven remedies are harmless, but some aren't. And even a harmless one can hurt you if it causes you to stop or slow down treatments prescribed by your doctor.

Study this checklist to judge potential treatments with a critical eye:

Checklist for Evaluating New or Unproven Remedies

Is it likely to work for me? Suspect an unproven remedy if it:

- uses only case histories or testimonials as proof
- cites only one study as proof
- cites a study without a control group (a group of people who did not receive the treatment)
- studies people who are not like you (and/or the control and treatment groups were not similar in age, sex, disease severity, and so on.
- cites results that could have been caused by something else.

How safe is the treatment? What possible dangers may it have? Suspect an unproven remedy if it:

- comes without any directions for proper use
- does not list contents
- has no information or warnings about side effects
- is described as "harmless" or "natural"
- is a diet that eliminates any basic food or nutrient or stresses only a few foods.

How is it promoted? Suspect an unproven remedy if it:
- claims it is based on a secret formula
- claims it cures fibromyalgia
- is available only from one source
- is promoted only in the media, in books, or by mail order, rather than in a reputable, scientific journal.

Pain Gate "Closers"

On the other hand, you can safely use a number of pain-relieving methods that involve both physical and mental factors. Try these techniques to see which work best for you.

Heat and Cold Treatments

It's an old but effective remedy—apply heat or cold to the painful area to reduce pain and stiffness. Cold packs, which are especially good for acute pain, numb the sore area and decrease inflammation and swelling. Heat treatments relax your muscles and stimulate circulation. Try them both and see which works best for you. Remember to follow the advice of your physician or physical therapist carefully when using these methods, especially heat.

Safety Tips for Heat and Cold Techniques
- Use only on dry and healthy skin so the treatment will not irritate any skin condition present. Dry yourself thoroughly after bathing and before using a heat treatment.
- Protect the skin over any bone that is close to the surface of your skin. Place extra padding over the area to prevent burning or freezing.
- Treat each area for only 15 to 20 minutes at a time. Let your skin return to its normal temperature before another application.
- Put a towel between your skin and any type of cold or hot pack.
- After the treatment, check the area for any swelling or discoloration.
- Gently move the painful areas to reduce stiffness.
- Do not use an electric device unless it is UL (Underwriter's Laboratory) approved and in good repair.

HEAT AND COLD TREATMENT IDEAS

HEAT

- Soak in a warm bath, shower, Jacuzzi, or whirlpool. Give sore muscles time to absorb heat—stay in at least until your fingertips are wrinkly.

- Place a heating pad or hot water bottle on the painful area. Don't sleep with the heating pad on, though, because it could burn you.

- Use an electric blanket or mattress pad. Turn it up before you rise, to combat morning stiffness.

- Use flannel sheets. They feel warmer against your skin.

- Use a hot water bottle wrapped in a towel to keep your feet, back, or hands warm.

- Warm your clothes by placing them in the dryer for a few minutes before you get dressed.

- Place hot packs—towels soaked in hot water or gel-filled bags that are heated in water or in a microwave and covered with a dry towel—on painful areas. Be careful not to let the pack get too hot.

COLD

- Place a cold pack or ice bag on the painful area. You can buy one at the drugstore, or you can make one by wrapping a towel around a bag of frozen vegetables.

- If you have Raynaud's phenomenon (see Glossary), you probably shouldn't use cold treatment. Ask your doctor.

Exercise

It may sound surprising, but another key to coping with pain is following a gentle exercise program designed by your doctor or physical therapist. A program including flexibility and endurance exercises, such as water exercise or walking, will help relieve stiffness and give you an improved sense of well-being. Exercise is such a vital element in controlling the symptoms of fibromyalgia, it is covered in its own chapter. (See Chapter 10 for in-depth information.)

Topical Ointments and Massage

Massage can relieve muscle spasm and increase blood flow, bringing warmth to the sore area. You can massage your own muscles, or you can ask your doctor to recommend a professional who is trained to give massages. If your shoulders, elbows, wrists, or fingers are painful, you may not be able to give yourself a massage. Electric massage devices can assist with self-massage. Some have infrared heads that direct more heat to the painful areas.

When giving yourself a massage, use lotion or oil to help your hands glide over your skin. Menthol gels also provide a comforting tingle.

Here are some tips for safe massage:

- Stop if you have any pain.
- Don't massage an area that is very swollen or painful.
- If you use a menthol gel for massage, always remove it before using a heat treatment—you might burn yourself.
- If you get a professional massage, be sure the masseuse is licensed in massage therapy (LMT) or is a physical therapist. You might ask if your massage therapist has treated patients with fibromyalgia; if so, you may want to talk to a patient to find out if or how he or she benefitted from massage therapy. To find a professional massage therapist, contact your state or local association of registered massage therapists, or call your local hospital or medical society for a referral.

Proper Body Mechanics

Use good body mechanics to perform daily activities in ways that are less aggravating to painful areas. These body mechanics tips will help reduce pain:

Good Posture

Practice good posture. Good posture puts the body in the most efficient and least stressful position, protecting your neck, back, hips, and knees. Poor posture is more tiring and adds to your pain.

Standing

Use your entire body to stand correctly. Imagine a straight line connecting your ears, shoulders, hips, knees, and heels. Now unlock your knees, tighten your stomach muscles, and tuck your buttocks under. Hold your shoulders back, tuck your chin in a comfortable position, and stand with your feet apart and spread slightly, or with one a little in front of the other to keep your balance.

If standing for a long time becomes painful, then sit down. Both of these actions flatten your back and prevent slouching.

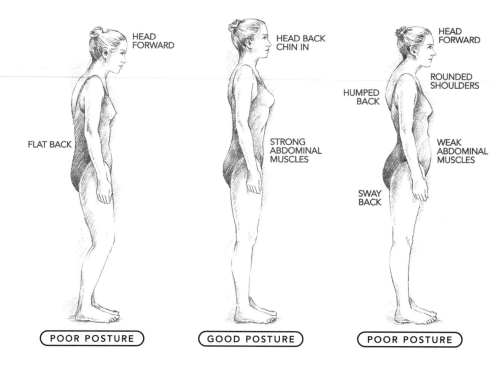

POOR POSTURE   GOOD POSTURE   POOR POSTURE

Good posture is defined as putting the body in the most efficient and least stressful position. Bad posture is more tiring and adds to your pain.

Sitting

Your spine should be stable and supported when you sit. To sit correctly: Use pillows or a rolled-up towel to support your lower back. Place your hips, knees, and ankles at a 90-degree angle (with a footrest, if necessary). Hold your shoulders back and tuck your chin in a comfortable position.

Your shoulders should be relaxed with your arms at your side, elbows at a 90-degree angle or lower, and your wrists straight. When working at a desk or counter, you may need to use an adjustable chair to position your joints for different work surfaces. Sit in a higher chair if it is difficult to sit down or stand back up. When reading, use a book stand to avoid neck strain when you look down.

Lying Down on Your Back

Sleep with a small rolled towel in your pillowcase or use a cervical (or neck) pillow to avoid stressing your neck or neck muscles.

Lying on Your Side

Try using several soft pillows or a large body pillow to support your arms and legs.

Body Leverage and Load Distribution

Lift or carry objects close to your body—it's less stressful. Slide objects whenever possible instead of lifting them.

Use your large, strong joints and muscles to lift or carry, and spread the load over stronger joints or larger surface areas. For example, carry a purse with a shoulder strap, bearing the weight on your larger shoulder joints to ease stress on elbows, wrists, and fingers. Or use a waist pack to eliminate stress on your lower back and improve posture. Use your palms instead of your fingers, and your arms rather than your hands, to lift or carry. When using stairs, go up with your stronger leg first and go down using your weaker leg first. Always use a handrail if available.

Movement

Staying in one position for a long time adds to stiffness and pain. Do a quick check of your jaw, neck, shoulders, arms, wrists, fingers, hips, legs, ankles, and toes. Stretch and relax areas that are tired or tight.

Weight Control

Extra pounds add stress to hips, knees, back, and feet, which can lead to further muscle strain. (Having just eight extra pounds is equivalent to carrying around a gallon of milk wherever you go.) If you are overweight, check with your doctor or nutritionist for advice about a weight-loss and exercise program. You'll look better, have more energy, and feel healthier. (See Chapter 11.)

Assistive Devices and Energy-Saving Techniques

Plan ahead, organize, and create shortcuts to save energy. The following common-sense tips for any busy person make even more sense for people with fibromyalgia:

- Combine errands and chores to get more done with less effort.
- Plan simple meals that require little preparation. Reheat leftovers

on microwave-safe plates (no pots and pans to wash!). On days you can spare the time and energy, cook extra portions to freeze.

- Don't be penny wise and pound foolish. Is driving an extra 15 minutes really worth saving 50 cents on groceries? Remember that your time and energy also have a value—as well as your gasoline. Try to keep shopping short and simple.
- Sit when you work, if possible. If not, take short rest breaks.
- Transport items on a cart whenever possible to avoid carrying them.

Use whatever alleviates stress from tired muscles. Helpful products can:

- provide leverage (e.g., lever faucets, tap turners, key devices, and doorknob extenders)
- extend your reach (e.g., long-handled items such as shoehorns, reachers, and bath sponges)
- save labor (e.g., electric can openers, pre-washed and -cut fresh vegetables, electric car windows, garage door openers).

Resources for Assistive Devices

Assistive devices are also known as self-help aids and devices, adapted equipment, and adaptive devices.

Organizations

The following organizations may have information about how to obtain assistive devices in your community:

- Arthritis Foundation
- Easter Seal
- Independent Living Center (The National Council on Independent Living [703/525-3406] has independent living centers in each state. Most centers have adaptive gadgets and devices for you to borrow at little or no cost for a trial period.)
- State Department of Vocational Rehabilitation
- Hospital physical or occupational therapy departments

Phone Book

If you want to buy devices, look in the Yellow Pages under the following headings:

- Hospital equipment and supplies
- Rental centers
- Pharmacies, drugstores

Hardware and Discount Department Stores

Shop by phone before leaving home. Ask if devices are actually stocked there or if you have to order them through catalogs. Compare prices.

Reference Books

Check your local library for books that contain suggestions on how to perform daily activities more easily. Some helpful titles are also listed in the Resources section of this book.

Positive Thinking

Because negative emotions can make your pain worse, your mind plays an important role in coping with illness. People with fibromyalgia who feel helpless and depressed about their condition have a tendency to decrease their activities, develop poor self-esteem, and feel worse. You can build a sense of control by adjusting your thoughts and actions.

Thinking differently may not get rid of your pain entirely, but having a more positive attitude can help. Try the following methods, and remember—practice and patience are required.

A Wellness Lifestyle

Having fibromyalgia can lead to a life built around pain and sickness. If you've been focusing on your illness, try devoting your attention to health instead. Live a wellness lifestyle. Think positively, indulge your sense of humor, enjoy a balanced diet, exercise regularly, and welcome activities with others. Follow your treatment plan, taking your medication properly, practicing relaxation techniques, and reaching out for help when you need it, whether from a doctor, therapist, or other professional. See Part Four of this book for more information on developing a wellness lifestyle.

Relaxation

Pain and stress have similar effects on the body. Muscles tighten, and breathing becomes fast and shallow. Heart rate and blood pressure rise. Relaxing can reverse these effects. It also endows a sense of control and well-being, making pain easier to manage.

Relaxation is more than just sitting down to read or watch TV. It involves learning to calm and control your body and mind. These skills don't come easily, especially if you are in pain. But practice helps. The best time to use relaxation skills is before your pain becomes too intense. Chapter 8 offers a full explanation of different types of relaxation techniques.

Distraction

Try taking your mind off pain by focusing on someone or something else. The more you concentrate on something outside your body, the less you will be aware of physical discomfort. Seek out engrossing interests—a new hobby, sport, computer game, book, or movie could help. Or help others by volunteering in your church or community.

Humor

Can laughter be the best medicine? Medical research suggests that its beneficial effects on mind and body are not easily dismissed, particularly when it comes to restoring health and fighting pain.

"Researchers continue to examine the physical, emotional and psychological changes which occur during mirthful experiences," says retired doctor William F. Fry Jr. of Stanford University Medical School in the April 1992 issue of the *Journal of the American Medical Association.* "These include physiologic activities involving the muscular, respiratory, cardiovascular, endocrine, immune and central nervous systems. In most cases, mirthful responses are positive and beneficial."

For people with pain, the most immediate merit of merriment may come about when it is used in the management of pain.

"If you can live with the pain, you can handle everything else, because pain is our worst symptom," says Bob G. McDaniel of Hot Springs, Arkansas, a certified instructor for the Arthritis Foundation's self-help, support group and aquatics exercise programs. "Laughter helps knock the edge off of it," says this veteran of osteoarthritis. "In fact, for me, the benefit ratio runs about 8:1—two hours of pain relief from 15 minutes of laughter medication."

Try these ideas to keep your humor quotient high.

- *Discover your personal humor preferences.* Just as each of us has different tastes in food and clothing, we also respond to different types of humor. Make it a point to observe and evaluate humor's heroes and heroines of the stage and page, both past and present. Seek them out in video marts, public libraries and bookstores and begin your own collection.
- *Keep a humor notebook.* Make a list of those comedians, cartoons, audiotapes and comedy movies that have the power to turn over your tickle box. Add your favorite comic strips, witty sayings, newspaper clippings, funny family stories and jokes. Carry it in your briefcase or keep it on your nightstand for regular reference and reading.
- *Share the fun.* Do certain friends, relatives or co-workers make it easy for you to relax and enjoy yourself? Make sure that having fun is a high priority when you spend time with them.

Remember the words of comedian-pianist Victor Borge: "The shortest distance between two people is a smile."

- *Cultivate an eye and an ear for humor.* Learn a tasteful, timely, funny joke every week and tell it. People will soon begin to swap their favorites as well. Watch for and create humor in everyday situations, particularly in times of stress, then write your observations down to share with others.

- *Decorate your home and office.* Ask friends and family to send you anything funny. Display these items on a bulletin board or refrigerator door where you can see and enjoy them often.

- *Get a good belly laugh going.* Set aside a time at regular intervals for the specific purpose of generating genuine laughter. Don't settle for a chuckle or two; focus on hearty, healthy howling.

- *Learn to laugh at yourself.* Everyone has flaws and shortcomings. Pick out several of your own and exaggerate them, poke fun at them. Then others will know you don't take yourself too seriously and will feel at ease when spending time with you.

*"Take a Laugh Break" by Janet R. Edwards, Corpus Christi, Texas, reprinted from **Arthritis Today**, January/February 1993.*

ACTIVITY: Create Your Own Pain-Management Plan

Now that you've read this chapter, you have some idea of how to control pain. Consider making a chart of your own pain-control methods. This will help you keep track of which methods work best for you. Adapt the work sheet on page 66 to your own purposes. Post it where you can refer to it often, such as on your refrigerator or medicine cabinet.

WORK SHEET: MY PAIN-MANAGEMENT PLAN

I take these medications at these times:_____

Name of medication:_____

Schedule:_____

_____

Heat, cold, or massage can help my pain. What I will do:_____

When will I do it:_____

Rest is important in managing my pain. I will rest:_____

_____

Exercise can help my pain and stiffness. I will do (types of exercises): _____

_____

I will do these exercises (how often/when):_____

Being calm and relaxed helps the pain. My ways to practice relaxation are:

_____

I will practice _____times each day.

Keeping my mind off the pain is important. When I'm in pain, I will think about (list some pleasant thoughts or memories):_____

I need to keep my life focused on healthful habits. One new healthful habit I'm going to practice is:

_____

I'm going to ask my doctor or therapist these questions about my treatment program:

_____

The following resources can help me:

Resources, address & phone nos:_____

Local Arthritis Foundation:_____

Local fibromyalgia organization:_____

Doctor:_____

Therapist(s):_____

Pharmacist:_____

Other members of my health-care team:_____

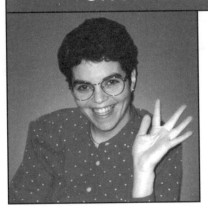

Mind Games
by Wendy Rivilis
Thiensville, WI

The next time your body is acting up, try one of these distractions. When you successfully divert attention from your aching muscles, you'll feel less pain. The brain, amazing though it is, can only process so much input at once. So practice your powers of concentration and see what a relief mind games can be.

Add a Dash of Drama—Envision a dramatic situation that uses the pain as part of the script. Pretend you're an actor playing a character in pain, a wounded spy escaping your captors or a sports hero taking your team to victory despite your injury.

Savor the Past—Conjure up the details of a favorite pain-free, pleasant moment from your past. Relive the good feelings of that time.

Challenge Yourself—Lose yourself in a game or project that requires your complete concentration. Try sewing, video games or solitaire, to name a few.

Smarten Up—Read a book or use instructional video or audiotapes to learn something new. Learn to paint; speak a foreign language; grow herbs; or delve into the spiritual practices of Native Americans or the juicy life of a celebrity.

Tune In—Listen closely to your favorite music. Soothing, absorbing music can be anything from classical to jazz or from gospel to Broadway show tunes.

Say Goodbye—Imagine pain leaving your body. Be creative and visualize the details. For example, picture mailing your pain away. See yourself scooping pain out of your body, placing it into a shipping carton, addressing the box to a faraway place and sending it off.

Get Competitive—Find a partner and play a word game, board game or card game.

Seek Nature—Enjoy the birds nibbling at your feeder or the fish swimming in your aquarium. Go into the woods or find a great mountaintop view.

Go to Neutral Territory—Compose your to-do list, mentally re-create the movie you saw last week, or come up with gift ideas for the holidays.

Call on Your Friends—Visit or phone friends and focus on someone else's life instead of your sore joints.

Help Others—Help others through a fibromyalgia support group or find some other way to focus your attention on others, not on yourself.

Reprinted from **Arthritis Today,** *November/December 1995. Wendy Rivilis is a freelance writer who has had degenerative disk disease for more than a decade. Her favorite distraction is her 3-year-old daughter.*

My Bowl of Marbles
by Linda Jean Frame

I begin by thinking of energy as marbles. Each small, expendable amount of energy becomes a marble. I have a limited number of marbles to use each day and while the number of marbles may vary from day to day, I can pretty well judge each morning just how many marbles I will have to use that day. I then place my day's supply in an imaginary fish bowl and begin my day.

With each activity—washing my face, combing my hair, etc., I use energy. When I expend one marble's worth of energy, I extract one marble from the bowl. (I value each marble at a certain amount and can judge when I use that amount of energy.) Bigger projects require more marbles; however, on bad days you will find that even small activities will demand the use of more marbles than those same activities will require on your good days. There are times when it is very frustrating to have so little energy and to have to use so much of it to do even simple things, but that's the way it is!

Starting each day with an awareness of your energy supply will enable you to choose what is really important to you, and you can plan accordingly. Remember that frustration is a form of stress and stress is a marble user! Remove marbles during the day for any type of stress, and for anything that causes tension or fear. For instance, I throw out a couple of marbles every time I have to drive in rush-hour traffic, because I know that I must be a little more alert and stressed than when I drive at other times of the day. If something happens to really stress me out, I may throw out the whole bowl of marbles and give myself the rest of the day off. If you should see me at one of those times when I have resigned from the human race, you might say, "Linda has lost her marbles!"—and you would be exactly right!

Linda Jean Frame, a former president of the Lupus Foundation of America, San Diego Imperial County Chapter, is deceased. This essay is reprinted with permission from "TALS," the San Diego Chapter Newsletter.

CHAPTER SIX

Coping with Fatigue

What Is Fatigue?

To healthy people, fatigue is usually caused by a few late nights or excessive physical exertion, quickly alleviated by a nap or a good night's sleep. For someone with fibromyalgia, however, fatigue can be an all-encompassing blanket of exhaustion. It may come and go, but sleep or rest do not restore a vigorous, alert state. In fact, sleep is of poor quality and perpetuates the feeling of tiredness.

Factors like sleep that affect fatigue are addressed elsewhere in this book. Getting a good night's rest is covered in Chapter 7; exercise, another essential treatment to restore energy, is covered in Chapter 10. Many pain-management techniques in Chapter 5 also battle fatigue—see tips on pain gate "closers" such as proper body mechanics, energy-saving, and assistive devices. The painful habits described in Chapter 5—smoking, drinking, and negative thinking—can also deepen fatigue.

Managing fatigue means walking a fine line between doing too much and doing too little. Many people with fibromyalgia push themselves so hard that they make themselves worse. Others surrender to the exhaustion and give up activity altogether. They, too, only increase their fatigue through inactivity.

This chapter is about finding the proper balance. You probably won't be able to eliminate your fatigue completely. But you can lessen it, by setting priorities and conserving your strength for what is most important to you.

Setting Priorities

To get a clearer idea of what is important to you, develop a "To Do" list. List everything you have to do during a typical week, and then rate how important each activity is. You might try a simple scale like: A = must be done; B = should be done; or C = could be done.

Look at your daily routine and responsibilities in light of your current energy level and then ask yourself these questions:

- What is most important to you personally? Think in basic terms of family, work, friends, church, hobbies.
- What activities are relevant to the priorities you've identified?
- What must you accomplish?
- What can you eliminate?
- What can you ask other people to do?
- What can be modified or simplified?
- What can you say no to? Sometimes this may mean saying no to yourself, as well as to other people.

A FEW WORDS ABOUT YES AND NO

If you find you're often too proud, too stubborn, or just don't have the heart to say no, study the following rules to help yourself get comfortable with that all-important two-letter word.

RULE #1: KNOW YOURSELF

Be honest with yourself about your limitations—only then can you effectively explain them to other people. Realize that you can't be all things to all people.

RULE #2: EXPLAIN YOUR ANSWER

When fibromyalgia forces you to say no, explain why. This helps educate family, friends and coworkers about your condition and helps them understand your limitations.

RULE #3: SPEAK GENTLY

When you're in pain, "no" doesn't always come out in the nicest way. Try to get your message across without bitterness or rancor.

RULE #4: BE HONEST WITH CHILDREN

Tell children in simple terms what you can and can't do and why. Then allow them their feelings of disappointment.

RULE #5: CHERISH THE YESES

When you finally learn to say no, it can be liberating. It allows you the energy to thoroughly enjoy each time you are able to say, "Yes!"

From "Learning to Say No" by Janice Hayes, **Arthritis Today**, *May/June 1996.*

Pacing Yourself

No matter how well you have prioritized, if you don't pace yourself properly, you may not have the stamina to carry out your plan. Estimate your energy level realistically, and allow for adjustments as your fibromyalgia worsens or improves. Here are some tips:

- Take breaks during or between tasks, before you get too tired. A ratio of 10 minutes of rest to every 50 minutes of activity works well for many. When your fibromyalgia is more active, rest longer and more frequently.
- Alternate light and heavy tasks, doing the toughest jobs when you're feeling your best. Stick to the time you'd planned to work and then quit—you'll get more done in the long run than if you wear yourself out.
- Avoid rushing. You'll be more efficient at a comfortable pace than on a hectic schedule that invites mistakes and accidents. Allow time for the unexpected.
- Divide big jobs into little ones.
- Avoid activities that tax you beyond endurance. For some people, that might mean the New York Marathon. For others, it's the monster truck rally your husband insists you'll enjoy. Just say no.

Problem Solving for Fatigue

In Chapter 3, tips are offered on how to approach problems creatively, using brainstorming and other techniques. The following examples below show how to use those methods on problems associated with fatigue.

In the example below, the problem is methodically analyzed. Use the numbered points to apply the same logic to your own sticky situations. Ask family and friends for suggestions when you get stuck.

PROBLEMS AND ALTERNATIVES

PROBLEM: Because of the pain and fatigue associated with your fibromyalgia, you are having difficulty maintaining your yard.

ALTERNATIVES: Consider other options that will help you achieve this task.

1 Change method or environment:

- Sit to do trimming.
- Use proper body mechanics.
- Hire a caretaker.
- Plan a patio garden of container plants rather than large beds.
- Move to an apartment or condominium where a groundskeeper provides lawn care.
- Work in small areas each day.
- Plant low-maintenance ground cover instead of grass.
- Have flower beds built at waist-high level to prevent stress on your back.

2 Use equipment:

- Use a self-propelled mower or a riding mower.
- Use long-handled trimming devices and weeding tools.
- Keep a stool nearby for rest periods.

3 Avoid heavy lifting:

- Use a cart to move equipment.
- Use lightweight equipment.

THE NEXT EXAMPLE ALLOWS FOR A MORE GENERAL APPROACH TO PROBLEM SOLVING.

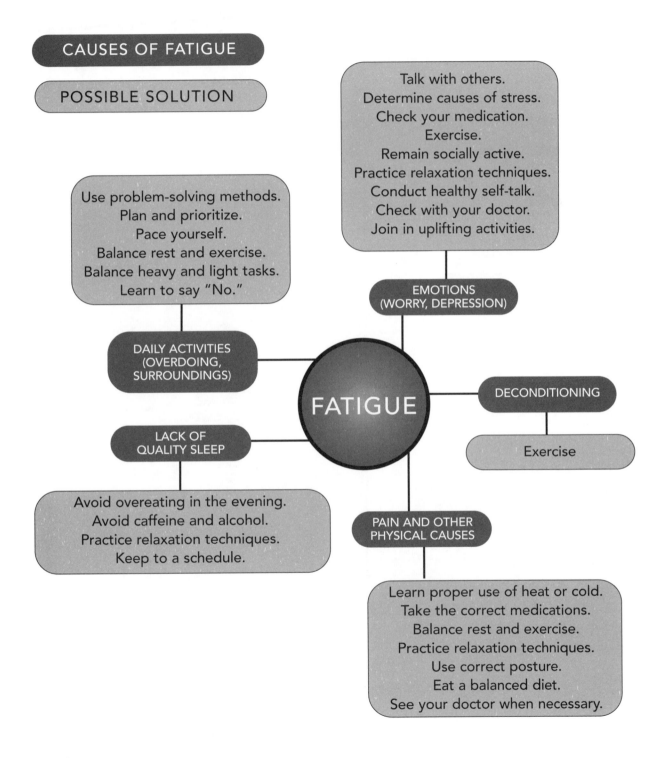

CAUSES OF FATIGUE

POSSIBLE SOLUTION

Talk with others.
Determine causes of stress.
Check your medication.
Exercise.
Remain socially active.
Practice relaxation techniques.
Conduct healthy self-talk.
Check with your doctor.
Join in uplifting activities.

Use problem-solving methods.
Plan and prioritize.
Pace yourself.
Balance rest and exercise.
Balance heavy and light tasks.
Learn to say "No."

EMOTIONS
(WORRY, DEPRESSION)

DAILY ACTIVITIES
(OVERDOING,
SURROUNDINGS)

FATIGUE

DECONDITIONING

Exercise

LACK OF
QUALITY SLEEP

Avoid overeating in the evening.
Avoid caffeine and alcohol.
Practice relaxation techniques.
Keep to a schedule.

PAIN AND OTHER
PHYSICAL CAUSES

Learn proper use of heat or cold.
Take the correct medications.
Balance rest and exercise.
Practice relaxation techniques.
Use correct posture.
Eat a balanced diet.
See your doctor when necessary.

Plan Your Own Course of Action Against Fatigue

Based on the examples on page 72 and 73 use the blank chart below to describe a probable cause of your fatigue, and then write down several possible options for dealing with it. Consider the advantages and disadvantages of each option, and then try one. After implementing the option selected, evaluate your results.

FATIGUE PROBLEM-SOLVING WORK SHEET

CAUSE OF FATIGUE	POSSIBLE SOLUTIONS

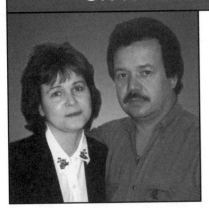

Thelma and her husband, Mike

The Importance of Resting
by Thelma Stone
Morgantown, WV

Like so many people, I often try to do too many things in one day and was usually able to get away with it until several years ago when I was diagnosed with fibromyalgia. Each daily activity took more effort than ever before and I pushed myself to exhaustion most of the time. In the beginning, I really thought that if I just kept on going as usual, my symptoms would go away. Instead, they just got worse.

Slowly, I came to realize that by allowing myself rest periods during the day the pain was less severe. It was very difficult to stop and take that break when there was still so much to be done, but I noticed that the tasks became a little easier after I had rested. Lying down when possible worked the best, but even sitting down and putting my feet up on something helped a lot. I found I was able to get through the day without the pain reaching that unbearable pitch that made me feel like I was falling apart and not accomplishing anything at all. Over the years, I have learned many ways to help reduce the amount of pain but I think this one is most important.

With the help of my understanding husband, a supportive family, and the right doctors, I have learned to accept the changes that fibromyalgia has brought into my life. True, it's not the same kind of life I was living before my diagnosis, but it is still a good one.

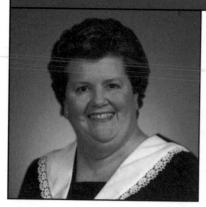

A Relaxing Night's Sleep . . . for a Change
by Delores Sisco
Huntsville, AL

As a person with a combination of arthritis conditions including rheumatoid arthritis and fibromyalgia, I find each day a challenge to get through. Because my pain was so intense, I often had trouble getting to sleep at night. Now, I have finally found a way to completely relax and get a good night's sleep. If you have fibromyalgia, you may want to give it a try yourself.

I have discovered that when you raise your arm, for example, you have to make an effort within your body to make it possible. This force is inside your body and only you can control it. If you can turn loose of this force—starting at your toes and working your way up your body—you will feel each muscle as it relaxes. As my muscles begin to relax, I can feel myself getting sleepy. I awaken the next morning more relaxed, refreshed, and rested than the night before.

What I have learned from this and from my doctor is that there is a force inside you that keeps these muscles tensed up and causes you to hurt more. All you need to do is let go of that force—and only you can do that. If you can successfully relax at night, you will find the next day easier to get through, something especially important in people with fibromyalgia.

The art of total relaxation is not an easy thing to accomplish. You have to work at it. I am not telling you that I am totally free of pain because it isn't so. Because my pain is so intense, I find that trying to relax my muscles at times does help a bit, but it especially helps at night when I'm trying to get to sleep.

CHAPTER SEVEN

Getting a Good Night's Sleep

Abnormal sleep patterns are a hallmark of fibromyalgia, and the culprits behind your fatigue. This chapter will give you a fuller understanding of your sleep problems and identify some ways to improve your sleep.

What Is Normal Sleep?

As essential to our bodies as breathing, sleep can be underappreciated in a 24-hour culture. But this basic of our daily life rhythms is vital to every dimension of health and well-being. Scientists are just beginning to discover its complexities. They've recently learned that sleep is not just a period of rest, but a time for certain critical bodily functions—among them, the release of hormones that are key both to sleep itself and to other purposes like healing and renewing tissue. We also now know that sleep is not the same experience for us throughout the night or throughout our lives.

Sleep is controlled by a primitive part of the brain—the hypothalamus—and occurs in stages. Stage 1 is a transition between wakefulness and sleep, lasting from about 30 seconds to several minutes. Stage 2 is the first level of true sleep. In Stages 1 and 2, the brain sends out faster-moving alpha waves which are a measure of brain activity. This is the stage in which sleepers spend most of their time; however, the deepest, most restorative stages of sleep occur later, in Stage 3 and Stage 4. In these stages, you're least likely to be awakened by an outside noise. A special, slow type of brain wave, called a delta wave, occurs only during this part of sleep, so Stages 3 and 4 are sometimes referred to as "delta sleep." Without delta sleep, you won't feel relaxed and refreshed in the morning.

Over the course of the night, you move in and out of the stages of sleep several times. If anything arouses you, you may awaken fully or partially. For example, you may be roused from deep sleep—but not fully awakened—if your spouse tumbles into bed after you are asleep. You may even mumble goodnight and exchange a kiss, still in Stage 1 sleep, then drift back to Stages 2, 3, and 4.

The stage of sleep during which you dream is known as REM sleep, so named because of rapid eye movements that occur under the closed lids during this phase. The first REM cycle of the sleep period normally occurs about 90 minutes after you fall asleep and lasts only five minutes. REM cycles occur approximately every 90 minutes during sleep. Psychologists and psychiatrists have long pondered the importance and meaning of dreams, but REM sleep may accomplish another important function: storage of information in long-term memory.

The amount of sleep needed differs greatly at various ages. Although we often hear that the average person needs about eight hours of sleep each night, scientists are finding that sleep requirements are highly individualized, determined by each person's biological clock. That need changes across your life span, as well as in keeping with events in your life, such as illness or injury.

An infant needs long stretches of sleep throughout the day. A small child needs one lengthy, sustained period during the night and at least one nap during the day. An adult usually needs one sustained period that is shorter than a child needs, although studies are showing that there are variations even on the "sustained" formula.

Some people can adapt well to having their sleep divided into segments during the day and night, but they still need delta sleep during those segments. Older people tend to awaken earlier, and awaken more easily to sound or other disturbances—but they never outgrow their need for delta sleep, and they tend to make up for the lesser amount of sleep during the night by drifting off to sleep during the day. As you'll see in our discussion below, interruption or lack of delta sleep is a key factor in the occurrence of fibromyalgia and its associated symptoms.

Fibromyalgia and Sleep

People with fibromyalgia often wake with the feeling that they haven't slept at all. In fact, they may have slept, but people with fibromyalgia tend to have a higher proportion of alpha-wave sleep than normal. In fact, alpha waves *intrude* on delta sleep in people with fibromyalgia, who in essence are roused again and again during the night. Consequently, they get considerably less delta sleep and are cheated of its restorative effects. They feel fatigued and sometimes overwhelmed by the need to nap.

Factors That Can Disturb Sleep

Begin by eliminating other factors besides fibromyalgia that may contribute to sleep problems. The following list will help:

Sleeping Pills

If used occasionally, sleeping pills can be helpful. However, if used nightly, they can produce an abnormal form of sleep, robbing you of REM. Without REM, you'll be deprived of dreams, a situation that eventually can cause nightmares. Also, sleeping pills can carry the side effects of a next-day "hangover" or grogginess, especially in older people who metabolize drugs more slowly. A newer sleeping pill called zolpidem tartrate (*Ambien*) may overcome some of these problems, as its effects only last for four to six hours and does not disrupt deep sleep. This medication should only be taken as prescribed by your doctor, who can take into account other medicines you may be taking.

Drugs and Foods

Many drugs can interfere with sleep. Steroids, which have many uses (including relief of inflammation of rheumatoid arthritis or lupus, relief of joint inflammation, and allergy relief), may cause sleep difficulties, especially if the dose is high. Cold medicines that contain antihistamines, headache medications that contain caffeine, and antidepressants (e.g. *Prozac*) are other causes of sleeplessness.

Caffeine in soft drinks, coffee, and tea can also cause problems. If you have trouble sleeping, try eliminating all caffeine from your diet, and review with your physician any drugs you are taking, including over-the-counter drugs such as diet pills, that may contain large doses of caffeine. Along with developing a progressive sensitivity to caffeine, older people may find that excessive sugar can also trigger sleeplessness.

Eating Habits

We are all familiar with the experience of lying awake at night after eating too much or eating the wrong kind of food. The resulting stomach distress can prohibit sleep. If you are lactose intolerant, drinking a glass of hot milk before bedtime is the worst thing you can do for your sleep. It's also important to avoid drinking excessive amounts of fluid before bedtime. If you have to get up in the middle of the night to urinate, you may then find it difficult to go back to sleep.

Smoking

Smoking is an unhealthy habit that's inadvisable for anyone. Some people say they smoke to relax, but in fact nicotine stimulates the nervous system. It only makes falling asleep more difficult.

Drinking

Alcohol, a depressant, can help you doze off initially, but you may awaken after the alcohol is metabolized and then have difficulty returning to a restful sleep. Thus, alcohol-induced sleep may only be short term, and the psychological and physical effects of alcohol-induced depression on people with fibromyalgia can make the condition worse.

Environment

Can you make your sleeping environment more conducive to rest? Address problems of excessive heat, cold, light, or noise, to make the most comfortable haven possible.

Stress

Stress can certainly hamper your ability to sleep. If you have recently gone through an upsetting experience, or if you take the day's problems to bed, it is difficult to relax. Stress in your home life or workplace can carry over into the bedroom by creating anxiety or excitement. Relaxation techniques used in the evening or before bedtime can help this problem. See Relaxation Tips and Techniques in Chapter 8.

It's a common problem in our society for people to work long hours and then lie in bed trying to forget about their job. This is especially defeating if you also engage in work-related activities in the bedroom. The bedroom should be a special room for rest and relaxation, and not an office or study.

Physical Problems

Any disturbing feeling—whether it's genuine pain or a little itch—can make it hard to sleep. People with fibromyalgia sometimes try to ignore their pain during the day, then at night find that it's impossible to ignore. If you have sustained pain (that is, any pain that is not fleeting) at any time, you should take your medications to keep it under control. If your physician has prescribed an anti-inflammatory drug, take it as prescribed, even when you feel better. A dose of your pain reliever at bedtime will work much better if you listen to your body and take care of it during the day, as well as at bedtime.

The ups and downs of hormonal fluctuations can also present challenges to sleep. Many women have trouble sleeping in the days before, during, or after their menstrual period. Pregnancy-related hormonal changes affect sleep patterns, especially in the first three months and the final month of pregnancy. Hot flashes and night sweats associated with menopause, when estrogen levels are low, may awaken a woman from a sound sleep or keep her from getting to sleep.

Nocturnal myoclonus is a benign type of muscle contraction that occurs at the onset of sleep. It has recently been recognized to be associated with fibromyalgia. It occurs as a twitch or sometimes vigorous jerk of the leg or legs. The problem may first be noticed by your sleep partner, but in any case, it interrupts the path to sleep. Myoclonus can be treated with a drug called clonazepam *(Klonopin)*, if necessary.

Another potential leg problem is restless legs syndrome, in which peculiar sensations in the legs provoke a need to move them. The sensations have been described as crawling, spastic, twitching, or painful, and they can cause repeated interruptions of sleep or inability to fall asleep. Your physician may prescribe tricyclic antidepressant drugs such as amitriptyline *(Elavil)*, which can help relieve this problem in most people. For more information on tricyclic antidepressants, see Chapter 2.

Some people have difficulty breathing when they sleep, which in turn keeps them from getting a restful night's sleep. In some cases, the problem occurs when airways become blocked during sleep. Called obstructive sleep apnea, this condition is best confirmed in a sleep laboratory by a physician experienced in this field. Since breathing difficulties occur more commonly in people who are overweight, weight reduction may be a solution. In addition, your doctor may recommend a continuous positive airway pressure device, or CPAP, to keep airways open while you sleep.

TIPS FOR IMPROVING YOUR SLEEP

- Maintain a regular daily schedule of activities, including a regular sleep schedule.

- Exercise, but not in the late evening.

- Set aside an hour before bedtime for relaxation.

- Eat a light snack before bedtime. You should not go to bed hungry, nor should you feel too full.

- Make your bedroom as quiet and as comfortable as possible. Maintain a comfortable room temperature. Invest in a comfortable mattress and/or try a body-length pillow to provide more support.

- Use your bedroom only for sleeping and for being physically close to your partner.

- Arise at close to the same time every day, even on weekends and holidays.

- Avoid caffeine (in coffee, tea, cocoa, soft drinks) and alcohol before bedtime.

- Avoid long naps. If a nap is needed to get you through the day, keep it short and schedule it well in advance of your bedtime. Try exercising in the afternoon rather than napping.

- Avoid sleeping pills.

- Don't smoke. If you must smoke, don't smoke before bedtime.

- Use a clock radio with an automatic shutoff to play soft music at bedtime. If you are not a heavy sleeper, wake up to music rather than a clanging alarm.

- Take a warm bath before going to bed.

- Listen to soothing music or a relaxation tape.

- Read before bedtime if you like, but avoid suspenseful, action-filled novels or work-related material that can preoccupy your thoughts and cause a poor night's sleep.

- Use earplugs or white noise to block distracting noises.

- Before going to bed, write down your worries and make a "Things to Do" list. Then put it away for tomorrow so you can stop thinking about them.

- If you don't go to sleep within the first 30 minutes after going to bed, or if you wake up in the middle of the night and can't get back to sleep, get up and go to a different room. Try a relaxation technique, read, or listen to soothing music.

CHAPTER EIGHT

Mastering Stress

What Is Stress?

By definition, stress is the body's physical, mental, and chemical reactions to frightening, exciting, dangerous, or irritating circumstances. Too much stress can worsen the symptoms of fibromyalgia.

Stress is a normal part of life. Many situations can be stressful, such as a move to a new town, a change in jobs, divorce, or the death of someone close to you. But stressful events are not always what you might consider to be negative. Weddings, births, and vacations are happy occasions that can also be nerve-racking.

Dealing with stress is a daily challenge. By learning to control your stress, you can reduce your pain, feel healthier, and manage your condition more effectively.

People with fibromyalgia go through the same kinds of stressful periods as everyone else. However, having a chronic health condition can add a new set of challenges and daily adjustments. You may have to rely upon family members and health-care professionals more than in the past. You may have to alter your lifestyle or give up favorite activities because of limited abilities. None of these changes is easy—and all can be upsetting. It's important to learn how to understand and manage your stress so these adjustments will be easier to handle.

Positive Stress Versus Negative Stress

Stress is supposed to be a temporary response, a sort of "emergency setting" that revs our engines and shifts us into high gear. But if you get stuck on that setting, stress becomes unhealthy. Here are some differences between positive/healthy and negative/unhealthy stress reactions:

Healthy stress is followed by relaxation. Your perceived resources balance out your perceived demands. After you've dealt with the situation, your body returns to its pre-stressed state—heartbeat and breathing

ON A PERSONAL NOTE

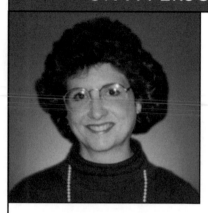

Take an Indulgence Break
by Annette Shelton
Monroe, LA

To cope better with fibromyalgia, I have chosen to allow myself to indulge in many simple pleasures throughout the day. I work on necessary tasks no more than one or two hours without an indulgence break. By generously sprinkling every day with activities in which I find pleasure, the pain, though still there, recedes into the background of my conscious thoughts.

A break of 10 to 15 minutes is all it takes to help me feel better. Here are some suggestions for indulging yourself:

- Have a pet—they love to cuddle, play, and lick tears.
- Sit on the porch with a cup of coffee and enjoy whatever is in sight.
- Read a psalm or poem or write a note to a friend.
- Take a walk and pay special attention to wildflowers, birds, and plants along your route.
- Play the piano and sing as loudly as you want.
- Call a friend to chat.
- Keep a crossword puzzle, jigsaw puzzle, or other brainteaser handy.
- Do gentle stretches and range-of-motion exercises to the tune of your favorite upbeat music.
- Keep a hobby to work on or a collection to look at while you rest.

*Reprinted from **Arthritis Today**, March/April 1996.*

slows, blood pressure goes down, muscles untense, and so forth. Your physical and emotional energies recharge, so that you can meet the next challenge.

Unhealthy stress occurs when your perceived demands exceed your perceived resources. You stay "geared-up" and don't relax. Your body is still in a stressed state—heart racing, blood pressure up, muscles tight, palms sweaty, stomach knotted. Because you aren't relaxing, your body and mind are unable to recover energy and balance, so the next challenge is difficult to meet. With each challenge, your physical and emotional resources become more exhausted. The stress has become chronic. Chronic stress can cause many negative effects on your body and mind. (See Table on following page).

EFFECTS OF CHRONIC STRESS

- headaches
- stomach distress, ulcers
- high blood pressure
- muscle tension, back pain and other types of pain
- chronic fatigue
- restlessness, irritability, frustration
- decreased zest for life, worry, fear, depression
- decreased performance and efficiency
- difficulty in making decisions, forgetfulness
- increased use of alcohol, cigarettes, or drugs
- eating and sleeping problems
- disease flares
- poorer immune function

How Does Your Body React to Stress?

When you feel stressed, your body becomes tense. This muscle tension can increase your pain. The increased pain can make you feel helpless and frustrated because it may limit your abilities. This can cause you to become depressed. A cycle of stress, pain, limited/lost abilities, and depression may develop. If you understand how your body reacts physically and emotionally to stress and learn how to manage stress, you can help break that destructive cycle.

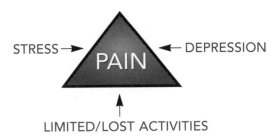

Stress, depression, and limited/lost activities can all contribute to pain.

Physical Changes

Some of your body's reactions to stress are easy to predict. At stressful times, the body quickly releases epinephrine chemicals into your bloodstream. This sets into motion a series of physical changes called the fight-or-flight response. These changes include a faster heartbeat and breathing rate, higher blood pressure, and increased muscle tension.

These physical changes give the body added strength and energy. They prepare your body for dealing with stressful events such as giving a speech or aiding an accident victim. When stress is handled in a positive way, the body restores itself and repairs any damage caused by the stress.

At times, you may feel unable to deal with stress in a positive way. As a result, stress-related tension builds up, and with no outlet, takes its toll on your body. This toll can take many forms—headaches, upset stomach, or worsened fibromyalgia symptoms. New research shows that stress may affect the body's immune system, leading to illness, fatigue, or other physical problems. Researchers haven't yet pinpointed how stress affects the immune system, but studies to solve the mystery are under way.

Emotional Changes

Your mind's reaction to stress is harder to predict than your physical reaction. Emotional reactions vary, depending on the situation and the person. They may include feelings of anger, fear, anxiety, helplessness, loss of control, annoyance, or frustration. A small amount of stress can actually help people perform their best—during an exam or athletic event, or on stage. Under too much stress, people may become accident-prone, commit errors, and perform clumsily.

Each person may respond to stress differently. You may like to be busy, or you may prefer a slow pace with less activity. What you find relaxing may be stressful to someone else.

Problem Solving for Stress

The key to managing stress is to make it work for you instead of against you. Consider the following steps to a complete program for managing your stress:

- Recognize your body's stress signals.
- Identify what causes your stress.
- Change what you can to reduce stress.
- Manage or accept what you can't change.
- Adopt a lifestyle that builds resistance to stress.

Diagnosing Your Stress Symptoms

Remember that the definition of stress is a personal matter—a situation that is stressful for one person may be a pleasant event for another. The same is true for how stress affects us physically and emotionally. One person's stress is manifested by headaches and tight shoulder muscles. Another person seldom gets headaches but always gets an upset stomach.

Stress symptoms are often obvious, but not always. For example, a stress headache may begin as a slightly aching neck that you ignore (it doesn't really hurt, you tell yourself) until it turns into a pounding headache. Or, you may assume that digestive upset was caused by something you ate—until you notice the same thing happens every time you confront a stressful situation. By "listening" to your body, you can learn how stress affects you personally. (See Table below.)

LISTENING TO YOUR BODY

LISTENING FOR	SOME WARNING SYMPTOMS
HEADACHES	tight shoulder, arm, or neck muscles hunched shoulders clenched teeth
DIGESTIVE UPSETS	stomach knot or butterflies stomachache appetite loss diarrhea or constipation
EMOTIONAL REACTIONS	anxiety moodiness anger hopelessness low self-esteem poor concentration depression
SLEEPING PROBLEMS	trouble falling asleep waking up early, being unable to fall asleep again oversleeping, sleeping too much disturbing dreams
OTHER SIGNS	chronic fatigue cold, clammy hands heart pounding chest feels tight or heavy dry mouth

Identifying the Causes of Your Stress

What causes you the most worry and concern? What situations leave you anxious, nervous, or afraid? Learning what causes stress is a personal discovery—what causes stress for you may not bother someone else. Once you know what the stressful aspects of your life are, you can decide how to change them or adapt to them.

ACTIVITY: Keeping a Stress Diary

Record the events in your life that cause stress, as well as any physical or emotional symptoms that result. After one week, look for patterns in symptoms and what caused them and make life adjustments. Try to stop stress *before* it becomes a problem.

SAMPLE STRESS DIARY

DATE	CAUSE OF STRESS	TIME	PHYSICAL SYMPTOMS	EMOTIONAL SYMPTOMS
4/18	getting kids off to school	7 am	fast heartbeat, tightness of neck	feel rushed, disorganized
4/18	stuck in traffic	8:30 am	headache, heart beating faster, legs aching	frustrated, angry at being late
4/18	meeting presentation	10 am	fast heartbeat, dry throat, clammy palms	anxious, nervous

STRESS DIARY

Keep a diary or chart if you can and record the causes of your stress as well as physical or emotional symptoms you experience. Keeping a stress diary can help you learn what causes your stress and how you can avoid it.

DATE	CAUSE OF STRESS	TIME	PHYSICAL SYMPTOMS	EMOTIONAL SYMPTOMS

Changing and Managing the Causes of Stress

Once you've identified the causes of your stress, determine which stressful situations can be changed and which can't. Take action to change what you can control. Here are some strategies:

- Set goals and develop a plan of action for reaching them. Remember to include hobbies and friends in your planning. Delegate responsibilities when possible. Because of your fibromyalgia, be flexible about the time needed to complete a goal.
- List your priorities. What needs to be done immediately? What can be done later? What can be eliminated? You may need to buy groceries today, but you can wash the clothes tomorrow.
- Reduce as many daily hassles as you can. If rush-hour commuting bothers you, map out a new way to work—a longer one, if necessary—to avoid high-traffic areas. Has anyone really noticed or rewarded your overwork commensurate with your loss of health? It's likely that the company will still survive even if you scale back your hours. If certain people or places annoy you, avoid them. If you have to put up with them, decide at the outset that you won't allow them to get on your nerves. Use the Hassles Scale on page 91 in this chapter to identify stressful situations in your life.
- Aim to have more uplifting activities than hassles in your life. Use the Uplifts Scale on page 92 to rate how you're doing.
- When making a decision, ask yourself, "Does this take care of, or work for, me?" It's easy, perhaps especially for women, to become caught up in caring for others at the expense of your own health. Take time to pamper yourself and do things you enjoy.
- Plan ahead for special events so you can enjoy them rather than collapse from stress. Shop early or year-round for Christmas, Hannakuh, or birthday gifts so you won't be caught in a last-minute crush. Buy many cards at once—for birthdays, weddings, new babies, and anniversaries—so you'll have them on hand for occasions, rather than going out for one card at a time. If you're entertaining, decide realistically what food you can cook easily, and then buy the rest. Or make it a potluck bash.
- Use the Holmes Scale on page 93 in this chapter to help you identify major life events.
- Learn to say no without feeling guilty. It's OK to let other parents help your child's teacher with their class trip to the zoo. Turning down extra duties even for a short period of time can reduce your stress.
- Think "win/win" when resolving conflicts. Seek solutions that will benefit both sides. If you want to go for a walk and your spouse has chores to do, help finish the work and go walking together.

WORK SHEET: HASSLES SCALE

Hassles are irritations that can range from minor annoyances to fairly major pressures. Listed here are a number of ways in which a person can feel hassled. Go through the list and put a check by those hassles that have happened to you in the past <u>month</u>. (**Optional**: Rate how severe each hassle has been on a scale of 1-3 (1 = somewhat severe; 2= moderately severe; and 3 = extremely severe). Then, add up your total score. Compare to the score on your *Uplifts Scale* (See page 92). Aim for getting an Uplifts score that is at least twice your total Hassles score.

	✓	#		✓	#
1. Misplacing things			23. Not getting enough sleep		
2. Trouble with neighbors			24. Problems with your children		
3. Social obligations			25. Problems with your parents		
4. Health of family member			26. Problems with your spouse or lover		
5. Concerns about debts					
6. Smoking too much			27. Too much to do		
7. Drinking too much			28. Work unchallenging		
8. Trouble relaxing			29. Legal problems		
9. Trouble making decisions			30. Concerns about weight		
10. Problems with people at work			31. Not enough energy		
11. Customers or clients giving you a hard time			32. Feeling conflict over what to do		
			33. Not enough time for family		
12. Home maintenance			34. Property, investments, taxes		
13. Concerns about job security			35. Yardwork		
14. Don't like current job			36. Concerns about news		
15. Bored			37. Crime		
16. Lonely			38. Traffic		
17. Fear of confrontation			39. Pollution		
18. Illness			Other hassles not mentioned yet:		
19. Physical Appearance			40.		
20. Problems at work			41.		
21. Car trouble			42.		
22. Rising prices			43.		

UPLIFTS SCALE

Uplifts are events that make you feel good. They are sources of your contentment, satisfaction and joy. Put a check by any events that may have made you feel good in the last <u>month</u>. (**Optional**: Rate how <u>strongly</u> you feel that each of the following uplifts <u>improves</u> your spirits on a scale of 1 to 3 (1 = somewhat strongly; 2 = moderately strongly and 3 = extremely strongly). Then add up your total score. Compare to the score on your *Hassles Scale*. Aim for getting an Uplifts score that is at least twice your total Hassles score.

	✓		✓
1. Getting enough sleep		23. Spending time with family	
2. Being lucky		24. Buying things for yourself or your house	
3. Saving money			
4. Not working		25. Home pleasing you	
5. Having a pleasant conversation		26. Giving or getting a present	
6. Feeling healthy		27. Traveling	
7. Being with children		28. Doing yardwork	
8. Visiting, phoning or writing someone		29. Making a friend	
9. Relating well with your spouse or lover		30. Getting unexpected money	
10. Completing a task		31. Dreaming	
11. Being efficient; meeting responsibilities		32. Pets	
		33. Children's accomplishments	
12. Cutting down on smoking		34. Things going well at work	
13. Cutting down on drinking		35. Making decisions	
14. Losing weight		36. Confronting someone	
15. Good sex		37. Being alone	
16. Friendly neighbors		38. Knowing your job is secure	
17. Eating out		39. Feeling safe in your neighborhood	
18. Having plenty of energy		40. Fixing something	
19. Using drugs or alcohol		41. Meeting a challenge	
20. Relaxing		42. Flirting	
21. Having the "right" amount of things to do		Other uplifts, not mentioned yet:	
		43.	
22. Good times with friends		44.	

WORK SHEET: HOLMES SCALE

Check all the items that happened to you in the past year or that you expect to occur in the near future.

		✔			✔
1.	Death of a spouse 100		23.	Son or daughter leaving home 29	
2.	Divorce 73		24.	Trouble with in-laws 29	
3.	Marital separation 65		25.	Outstanding personal achievement 28	
4.	Jail term 63		26.	Spouse begins or stops work 26	
5.	Death of a close family member 63		27.	Begin or end school 25	
6.	Personal injury or illness 53		28.	Change in living conditions 25	
7.	Marriage 50		29.	Change in personal habits 24	
8.	Fired from job 47		30.	Trouble with boss 23	
9.	Marital reconciliation 45		31.	Change in work hours or conditions 20	
10.	Retirement 45		32.	Change in residence 20	
11.	Change in health of family member 44		33.	Change in schools 20	
12.	Pregnancy 40		34.	Change in recreation 19	
13.	Sex difficulties 39		35.	Change in church activities 19	
14.	Gain of new family member 39		36.	Change in social activities 18	
15.	Business readjustment 39		37.	Small mortgage or loan 17	
16.	Change in financial state 38		38.	Change in sleeping habits 16	
17.	Death of a close friend 37		39.	Change in number of family get-togethers 15	
18.	Change to different line of work 36		40.	Change in eating habits 13	
19.	Change in number of arguments with spouse 35		41.	Vacation 13	
20.	Large mortgage 31		42.	Holidays 12	
21.	Foreclosure of mortgage or loan 30		43.	Minor violations of the law 11	
22.	Change in responsibilities at work 29			TOTAL	

The scale shows the relative weights for stress-producing situations. Add up your score. If your score is between:

0—199=LOW STRESS   200—299=MEDIUM STRESS   OVER 299=HIGH STRESS

If your score is high, try to think of ways to decrease your score—can you eliminate or postpone some changes?

If You Can't Change the Situation, Change Your Outlook

You can only change yourself, not other people. Some situations can't be changed, but your point of view can. Try to roll with the punches. Being flexible helps you keep a positive attitude, despite hardships. Here are some ways to help you change your outlook.

- *Think positively.* Ask yourself if there is any hidden benefit to the stressful situation, and make the most of it. Getting fired or laid off from a job could lead to a spiral of depression, debts, and debilitating pain. Or it could be the opportunity you've been looking for to change your work situation for the better.
- *Run a reality check.* Try to evaluate the situation's real importance. Your daughter didn't call this week. Does it mean she's ignoring you, or that her own schedule was difficult to manage? And will your world collapse because she didn't call?
- *Develop and use support systems.* Share your thoughts with family, friends, clergy, or others who are good listeners and can help you see the problems in a constructive way. However, don't whine to others constantly about every detail of your discomfort. You may alienate your support structure and isolate yourself from the help you need, and you may be reinforcing your own bad habit of focusing on your pain.
- *Refocus your attention positively.* Thinking about something or someone else besides yourself can help you relax and distract you from pain.
- *Develop "safety-valves."* Release stress by literally working it out with exercise or by writing in a journal to process it.
- *Have fun.* Schedule time for play, and join activities that make you laugh. See Chapter 5 for more about the healing qualities of humor.

REALITY CHECK

LEARN TO PUT STRESSFUL SITUATIONS IN PERSPECTIVE BY ASKING THESE QUESTIONS.

- Does this situation reflect a threat signaling harm, or a challenge signaling an opportunity?
- Are there other ways to look at this situation?
- What exactly is at stake?
- What is the worst that can happen?
- What are you afraid will occur?
- What evidence do you have that this will happen?
- Is there evidence that contradicts this conclusion?
- What coping resources are available?

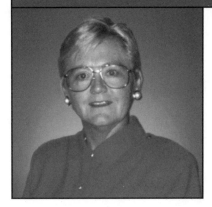

Getting Your Priorities Straight!
By Louise C. Pattison
Laveen, AZ

As a person—not a patient—with chronic pain, each activity, thought, and plan has a direct effect on how well I cope with the pain. If I allow my worries and responsibilities to escalate, my stress level increases and so does the pain. I have learned to set priorities, alleviating anger, resentment, and frustration.

I am—or was—a people pleaser, but through a slow mind-altering process, I gradually acknowledged my needs and the obligation to meet those needs first. If I ignore those needs, I'll eventually collapse. I'll be of no use to myself or anyone else. I have to realize that I can't give what I don't have any longer. It may take more time to do the simplest of tasks, but oh well, who cares—we have the time, don't we?

Every day, ask yourself: "What is of most importance to me today?" Keep a list—not only of problems—but also of those things that make you happy. The purpose of setting priorities is to realize that nothing is absolutely black and white, including your life. You must be flexible to learn to focus on your life instead of on your pain.

Set realistic goals—desires that can be reached—one step at a time. Become more assertive. Recognize your basic rights. Make mistakes. Say "No" sometimes. And ask questions. There are no wrong feelings. Begin to help yourself.

Relaxing to Reduce the Effects of Stress

Learning how to relax is one of the most important ways to cope with stress. Relaxation is more than just sitting back and being quiet. It is an active process, requiring practice, to calm your body and mind. Once you know how, relaxing becomes second nature. As you learn new methods, keep these principles in mind:

- Stress has many causes, which means there are many solutions. The better you understand what causes your stress, the more successfully you can manage it.
- Not all relaxation techniques will work for everyone. Whatever works for you is what's important. Try out different methods until you find one or two that you like best. You may learn that some techniques work well for certain situations, while others work better at other times.
- Remember that learning these new skills will take time. Practice new techniques for at least two weeks before you decide if they work well for you.

If you need help learning how to relax, see a mental-health professional or contact your local Arthritis Foundation chapter. A few common techniques for relaxing are described below, as well as several relaxation activities. See the Resources section of this book for information on audiocassettes you can purchase to accompany these activities.

Relaxation Tips
- Pick a quiet place and time of day when you won't be disturbed for at least 15 minutes.
- Make yourself as comfortable as possible before beginning. Loosen any tight clothing and uncross your legs, ankles, and arms. Sit in a comfortable chair or lie down.
- Try to relax daily or at least four times a week.
- Don't expect immediate results. It may be several weeks before you reap benefits from some techniques.
- Relaxation should be enjoyable. If these techniques are unpleasant or make you more nervous and anxious, stop. You may manage your stress better with other techniques.

ACTIVITY: Deep Breathing

Deep breathing is a basic technique that applies to almost all relaxation exercises. This simple technique is key to mastering the art of unwinding. Here are the steps:

1. Get as comfortable as you can—-loosen any tight clothing or jewelry, uncross your legs and arms. Close your eyes.

2. Place your hands firmly but comfortably on your stomach. This will help you feel when you are breathing properly. When you breathe correctly, your stomach expands out as you breathe in and it contracts in when you breathe out. (Many people breathe "backwards"—they tighten their stomachs when they breathe in, and relax their stomachs when they breathe out. If you're a "backwards breather," take a minute to get yourself coordinated.)

3. Inhale slowly and deeply through your nose to a count of three. Feel your stomach push against your hands? Let it expand as much as possible as you fill your lungs with air.

4. When your lungs are full, purse your lips (as if you were going to whistle) and exhale slowly through your mouth for a count of six. (Pursing your lips allows you to control how slow or fast you exhale.) Feel your stomach shrink away from your hands?

5. When your lungs feel empty, close your mouth and begin the inhale-exhale cycle again.

6. Repeat the inhale-exhale cycle three or four times at each session.

7. Whenever you're ready, slowly open your eyes and stretch.

Tip: Breathing deeply can make you feel light-headed or dizzy—especially when you are tired or hungry. It's a good idea to first practice deep breathing while you are sitting or lying down. Once you get the hang of it, deep breathing can be used anytime, anyplace.

ACTIVITY: Relaxation to Control Pain

Beginning Part (excerpted from "Imaginative Progressive Relaxation" technique):

First take some time to make sure that you are in a really comfortable position. Make a quick check from head to toe to determine whether your whole body is being supported. Adjust any parts that feel uncomfortable. Try not to have legs or arms crossed, but most importantly, do what is comfortable for you.

Now, close your eyes. Become aware of your breathing. Feel the movement of your body as you breathe in and out. Breathe in slowly and exhale. On your next breath, focus on the image of breathing in good, clean air . . . and exhaling all your tensions with your breath out. Allow your breathing rhythm to pleasantly slow down. Feel as though tension is being released each time you breathe out.

Middle Part:
Option 1: "Pain Drain"

Now, feel within your body and note where you experience pain or tension. Imagine that the pain or tension is turning into a liquid substance. This heavy liquid flows down through your body and out through your fingers and toes. Allow the pain to drain from your body in a steady flow. Now, imagine that a gentle rain flows down over your head . . . and further dissolves the pain . . . into a liquid that continues to drain away. Enjoy the sense of comfort and well-being that follows.

Option 2: "Disappearing Pain"

Now, notice any tension or pain that you are experiencing. Imagine that the pain takes the form of an object . . . or several objects. It can be fruit, pebbles, crystals, or anything else that comes to mind. Pick each piece of pain, one at a time, and place it into a magic box.

As you drop each piece into the box, it dissolves into nothingness. Now, again survey within your body to see if any pieces remain, and you may remove them if you wish. Imagine that your body is lighter now, and allow yourself to experience a feeling of comfort and well-being. Enjoy this feeling of tranquility and repose.

Option 3: "Healing Potion"

Now, imagine you are in a drugstore that is stocked with bottles and jars of exotic potions. Each potion has a special magical quality. Some are of pure white light, others are lotions, balms, and creams, and yet others contain healing vibrations. As you survey the many potions, choose one that appeals to you. It may even have your name on the container. Open the container and cover your body with that magical potion. As you apply it, let any pain or tension slowly melt away, leaving you with a feeling of comfort and well-being. Imagine that you place the container in a special spot and that it continually renews its contents for future use.

Option 4: "Leaving Pain Behind"

Imagine that you are dreaming now. Although your body stays in the same position, imagine that you are gently leaving it. . . . As you leave your body, notice that you have also left your tension and pain behind. Pick a special spot to visit, one that brings pleasure and a feeling of well-being. Notice how your dreamlike body feels as you visit this special place. Linger here for awhile . . . and when you feel ready, return to your position in alignment with your body. When you open your eyes, retain the freedom from tension and pain, and continue to experience a sense of comfort and well-being.

End Part:

Whenever you are ready, slowly stretch and open your eyes.

Adapted from *The ROM Dance,* a range-of-motion and relaxation program, Diane Harlowe and Patricia Yu, 1992. Materials available from The ROM Dance, P.O. Box 3332, Madison, WI 53709. (800/488-4940)

Guided Imagery

Think of guided imagery as a daydream with a tour guide. By diverting your attention away from stress, guided imagery takes your mind on a mini-vacation. Use your imagination to transport yourself to a more peaceful place. It's up to you to choose where. For some people the most relaxing place is the seashore; for others it's the mountains. Pick your mind's ideal vacation spot, and go there.

ACTIVITY: Guided-Imagery Smorgasbord

The following exercise teaches you how to focus on relaxing in your choice of desirable, stress-free locations. Again, have a friend read the exercise to you— or record it yourself and play it back as you imagine.

Beginning ritual:

Get as comfortable as you can, feet slightly apart, arms resting at your sides. Now close your eyes. Take a slow deep breath in through your nose and slowly exhale through your mouth. Again, take a deep breath in . . . and slowly exhale. Continue to breath slowly and deeply . . . Notice yourself getting more and more relaxed. Let all your tension melt away.

Middle part:

Option 1: "Sea"

Your body is very heavy, at ease and warm. . . . Listen to your heart . . . it is beating steadily . . . and regularly. . . . As you listen to your heart . . . you feel its beat . . . in your whole body. . . . It feels as though you are on a boat . . . on a quiet calm sea . . . with the water lapping against the sides . . .

You're inhaling and exhaling like the waves. . . . They are gently rocking you. . . . The rocking continues in your mind . . . and as you rock . . . one after the other the negative emotions are dropping out of you . . . frustration . . . sorrow . . . depression . . . heartache . . . worries . . . resentment. . . . You feel serene and content . . .

You feel so wonderful you'd like the whole world to enjoy it with you . . . and out of the depths of your heart rises a great lightness . . . and you feel it flow in a continuous steady stream through your whole body . . . and all the time you feel lighter . . . and lighter . . .

Adapted from the *Arthritis Movement Workshop Leader's Manual,* Arthritis Foundation, Arizona Chapter.

Option 2: "Pine Forest"

Imagine in as much detail as possible that you are sitting comfortably in a chair or hammock in the middle of a beautiful pine forest. . . . Enjoy the fresh, cool, clean, fragrant air. . . . What a pleasure it is to breathe! . . . Imagine the gentle, cool breeze as it touches your skin.

You are sitting comfortably, feeling peaceful and calm. . . . As you casually look around, you are impressed by the beauty of the tall pine trees with their rich brown bark . . . and graceful feathery green branches. You notice the pinecones on the branches. . . . You watch the leaves of the aspen trees dancing in the wind. The ground interests you with its rich brown dirt covered with pine needles and leaves . . . and its robust, earthy aroma.

You hear birds calling . . . and a woodpecker at work in the distance. . . . You notice a small clearing in the forest. The clearing is covered with green grass and beautiful wildflowers of all types and colors. You see butterflies around the flowers. You are at peace in your pine forest, sitting comfortably, feeling relaxed and calm . . . appreciating the wonders of nature . . . and of being alive.

Adapted from the *Multiple Sclerosis Self-Help Course Leader's Guide* by Katalina McGlone, 1984.

Option 3: "Ocean Beach"

Imagine that you are at the ocean. . . . You are sitting comfortably on the beach under the shade of a large beach umbrella. . . . Feel the warm sand under you . . . and the warm, comfortable air around you . . . and the refreshing, soft breeze blowing through your hair. . . . Feel the warm moisture in the air upon your face. . . . Notice the smell of the ocean . . . Imagine how beautiful, brilliantly blue the sky is . . .

You're sitting on the beach . . . feeling calm . . . peaceful . . . relaxed . . . comfortable. . . . You are watching the waves . . . as they grow and break . . . mesmerized as they go in and out from the shore. . . . You can hear the thundering of the waves as they break. . . . The only other sounds are those of the seagulls. . . .

Notice how peaceful you feel . . . sitting on the beach . . . feeling in harmony with nature.

Adapted from the *Systemic Lupus Erythematosus Self-Help Course Leader's Manual,* Katalina McGlone, 1984.

Option 4: "Floating in Space"

Imagine you are standing on a mat in front of an elevator. The doors open, you step in and watch the numbers slowly change: 1, 2, 3, 4, 5, 6, 7, 8, 9, 10. The doors open, and you step out into deep, dark outer space. Feel yourself floating weightlessly, drifting, being very light. See the pure, velvety deep blue color of space all around you. Look at the earth, small and green-blue . . . Imagine stars and planets moving past you in the distance. Imagine yourself moving towards a space of diffuse white light, as bright and ethereal as a distant star . . . As you approach this light, it increases in size until you feel yourself surrounded by its glow. Being in the light, you feel that you are bathed in feelings of tranquility and well-being.

If disturbing thoughts or feelings enter your mind as you are in this place, allow them to pass by you, just as you imagine planets and stars passing by you on this voyage. Let these thoughts and feelings fade into the distance, leaving them behind you in the same way that you might imagine a comet disappearing over the horizon.

Enjoy the peaceful feelings of this place. . . . Slowly float out of the white light, imagining that it has filled your body and you are carrying it with you. Then float back past the stars and planets through the deep velvety blue-black space to the elevator. Step back in, see the doors close, watch the numbers change: 10, 9, 8, 7, 6, 5, 4, 3, 2, 1. The doors open and you are back on your mat. Feel your body on the mat.

Adapted from the *Arthritis Movement Workshop Leader's Manual,* Arthritis Foundation, Arizona Chapter.

Option 5: "Memory and Fantasy"

In this relaxation exercise, remember a past experience—or create a new one—with your imagination.

Imagine yourself in an environment where you feel secure, comfortable and relaxed. This can be a place you remember . . . a fantasy you are creating . . . or a mixture of memory and imagination. Simply experience whatever comes to you. Sometimes the environment will change during the exercise, and sometimes it will remain the same.

Place yourself in this environment and note how you are positioned . . . standing . . . sitting . . . or lying down. In this secure, comfortable, relaxed environment, look around you. Take in the panorama of colors, forms and textures. If you are outside or can see outside . . . note the season . . . time of day or night . . . and the weather. Look all around you . . . in front . . . behind . . . both sides . . . above . . . and below you. Look at the sky or ceiling . . . the ground or floor . . . in the distance . . . and up close. Are there other people here? Take in all you wish to see. What sounds come to you? Listen for sounds in the distance . . . up close . . . all around you. From what directions do the sounds come?

In this secure, relaxed and comfortable environment . . . is there anything that you can smell? If something to drink or eat presents itself . . . taste it fully and note its texture in your mouth. Is there anything or anybody you are touching? How does it feel? How does the environment around you feel physically . . . warm or cool . . . damp or dry? Do you feel movement in the air? How does it feel emotionally? . . . How do you feel inside in this environment?

Once again, take in the sights around you. . . . They may have changed. Note the sounds . . . smells . . . tastes . . . and sights. Focus on emotional feelings . . . the feelings inside.

Adapted from *The ROM Dance,* a range-of-motion and relaxation program, Diane Harlowe and Patricia Yu, 1992. Materials available from The ROM Dance, P.O. Box 3332, Madison, WI 53709. (800/488-4940)

Option 6: "Water Fantasy"

Imagine that you are immersed in water, perhaps in your bathtub. . . in a lake . . . swimming pool . . . or even a whirlpool bath. Imagine that the water is the perfect temperature . . . just warm enough so that every muscle in your body feels as supple and flowing as the very water itself. Experience the water flowing around and coming into contact with each part of you. As it does this, it melts away deeper levels of tension . . . leaving your whole body feeling cleansed and drained of all tension.

Let yourself stay in this wonderful water for awhile, all the time continuing to allow yourself to let go of deeper and deeper levels of tension . . . and allowing yourself to feel more and more relaxed.

Adapted from *The ROM Dance,* a range-of-motion and relaxation program, Diane Harlowe and Patricia Yu, 1992. Materials available from The ROM Dance, P.O. Box 3332, Madison, WI 53709. (800/488-4940)

End Part:

(Silence) . . . You may go back to this place whenever you want, simply by sitting quietly and remembering this place in as much detail as possible. . . . Whenever you are ready, move your fingers, wiggle your toes, and come back to this world feeling refreshed and invigorated.

Build Up Your Resistance to Stress

Stress can have a negative effect on your body. Taking good care of your body can help you build up resistance to stress. Ways to take good care of your body include:

- eating a balanced diet
- exercising
- avoiding drugs and alcohol
- getting enough rest and sleep
- saving energy by pacing your activities
- accentuating the positive. See Part Four, "Living Well with Fibromyalgia."

Incorporate the relaxation techniques you've learned in this chapter into your daily life and you'll reap rewards. Managing your stress—whether or not you have fibromyalgia—can lessen pain and increase health and happiness.

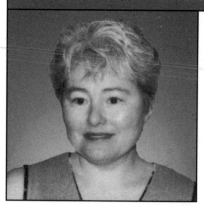

On a Personal Note: Less Is More
by Anne Makulowich Szymanski
Bethlehem, PA

Although our daydreams often remind us of the past when our energy knew no bounds, the reality of fibromyalgia is pain and fatigue. To adjust successfully to a chronic illness is to acknowledge ongoing limitations in our lives. However, in order to overcome self-defeat, we must also force ourselves to seek meaningful ways to express our new selves.

If overdoing my walk becomes an excuse to cancel daily exercise, then I can walk less distance each day but do it faithfully—and less is more.

If a morning of shopping overwhelms me, then I can add a roast chicken or hoagies to the grocery list for that night's supper. Tomorrow I might be able to prepare dinner as well as two other dishes to freeze for another time—and less is more.

If one medical appointment is all I can manage during the course of the day, then I can concentrate all my efforts to the best possible exchange of information and ideas that will help me over the course in the future—and less is more.

In other words, fibromyalgia has taught me over the course of 37 of my 47 years on earth, the inestimable need for patience and self-acceptance.

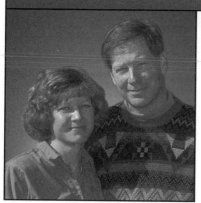

Sher and Gregg Piburn

Lightening the Load
by Gregg Piburn
Loveland, CO

As hip, young lovers in 1973, my wife Sher and I backpacked across the Continental Divide on our honeymoon. Our bodies were lean and muscular and we felt we could do anything.

But since that time, life has dealt Sher a difficult hand—the chronic condition of fibromyalgia that has forced her to redefine who she is. The physical aspect of her is now the weakest rather than the strongest part.

In the past, Sher and I would often head to the mountains for some cross-country skiing on Sundays. That's no longer possible due to Sher's health problems. For years, I stored my skis next to hers, making her illness as big a burden on me as it was on her. I was figuratively putting into storage a part of myself that gave me pleasure and confidence, creating a frustrated, miserable and angry man.

I finally had to grieve over the loss of the healthy Sher. One of the stages of grief is anger. I expressed my anger to a couple of good buddies and to my wife. When they heard my gut-level honesty about my own pain and frustration, they encouraged me to take better care of myself.

In fact, it is Sher herself who most often tells me to take a break, call a friend, and strap on the skis. While Sher wishes she could go, she also feels less guilt about her illness, knowing that I can still occasionally do physical activities that invigorate me.

I don't go skiing as much as I did early in our marriage, but the skis are out of storage and my attitude is far better than it was a few years ago. The load I carry is lighter now, and so is my heart.

*Reprinted from **Arthritis Today,** July/August 1996.*

CHAPTER NINE

Getting Past Grief and Depression

What Is Grief?

Chronic illness may change your life in so many ways it's hard to believe you're the same person. Little wonder then, that after the initial relief of diagnosis—of finally having a name for your problem—grief often sets in. Yet it catches many people by surprise.

Grief is a natural response to loss. Usually we think of grief in terms of death or divorce. Feelings of grief over the diagnosis of a chronic illness are not discussed very often, but that, too, involves loss.

For people with fibromyalgia, the losses are physical, social, and personal. Mourning these losses is not only natural, but necessary as part of a healing process that allows you to come to terms with the changes fibromyalgia has brought about. Giving yourself permission to grieve the loss of your old life will help you reach acceptance sooner. With acceptance, you can begin to build a new life.

Your spouse and family members may also need to grieve the changes in your health. Allow them to do it in their own way and in their own time.

POSSIBLE GRIEF RESPONSES

SHOCK AND DENIAL: "NO! IT CAN'T BE TRUE!"

Denial is a protective buffer, allowing you to replace anxious thoughts with more hopeful ones. This buys time for you to mobilize other coping techniques and face your losses at a manageable pace. This stage is usually temporary, but if you can't accept your diagnosis, you won't be able to fight your condition.

BARGAINING: "LET'S MAKE A DEAL."

You may find yourself making secret promises—for example, "I'll become a better person" if fate or a higher power sends a cure. Or you may begin an endless cycle of seeking other medical opinions and trying unproven remedies. This is yet another "time-buying" stage before acceptance.

ANGER: "WHY ME?"

Anger, rage, envy, and resentment are all common responses to bad news like a diagnosis of fibromyalgia. You may express your anger by criticizing your doctor, family, or friends. You may put off necessary chores or treatments, or sink into depression. You may feel cheated by fate or a higher power. But if you don't move beyond this stage, you can become extremely irritable and quarrelsome.

GUILT: "I DESERVED IT."

Next, you may blame yourself for having fibromyalgia. ("I should have been a better person; I should have taken better care of myself," and so on). You may begin to think of yourself as a burden to others, who you think find your illness repulsive. And just as you view your illness as a personal failure, you think if you try harder to do more, you'll feel better.

SADNESS AND DEPRESSION: "I WILL MISS BEING ABLE TO . . . "

This stage is a natural part of saying good-bye to lost roles and abilities. It usually gets better in time. However, if this stage persists, depression will set in as a lingering sense of despair and worthlessness. It can also be a quiet cover for anger, anxiety, or guilt. Depression persists until negative thinking is changed . . .

POSSIBLE GRIEF RESPONSES

FEAR AND UNCERTAINTY: "WHAT ELSE WILL HAPPEN?"

Also natural responses to fibromyalgia's unpredictable variations, fear and uncertainty themselves may cause muscle tension, increased heart rate, stomach distress, and trembling. Signs that you're stuck in this stage include anticipating the future with fear and anxiety, worrying about the next bad bout even during periods of good health, or feeling helpless or out of control over your health from day to day.

LONELINESS AND ISOLATION: "NO ONE UNDERSTANDS."

Curtailing your activities can lead to fewer social contacts. Also, some friends may withdraw because they don't know how to help. Family members may become emotionally exhausted. All these factors can lead to isolation and loneliness if you don't work at broadening your support system and maintaining contact with the outside world.

RECONCILIATION AND ACCEPTANCE: "I MAY HAVE FIBROMYALGIA BUT. . .

Acceptance is the final stage of grief, but the first sign you're ready to build a new life. Once you are able to let go of the past and the person you were before you developed fibromyalgia, you can get on with your recovery.

Grief's "Parade of Emotions"

Grief is a process made up of many feelings—a sort of parade of emotions. In her landmark book, *On Death and Dying*, psychiatrist Elisabeth Kubler-Ross, MD, described the stages of death that terminally ill people go through, and her description has been widely applied to mourning other losses.

However, the stages of grief rarely start at one point and proceed ahead in an orderly way until you reach the ultimate goal of acceptance. For most people, the grief process is more chaotic. You may not experience all these emotions, nor are you likely to experience them step by step. Your reactions may skip around, backtrack, or surge together simultaneously.

Grieving is a very personal process and each person proceeds through it at his or her own pace. How you move through grief depends to a great extent on your support systems and your basic personality. For example, if you have always been an outgoing person with a sunny disposition, you may not experience the anger or isolation that a more introverted person who has a quick temper may feel.

You also need to understand that grief can be ongoing. A worsening of your symptoms, the anniversary of a negative event, or being reminded of an activity that you can no longer participate in can provoke a reaction you thought you had put behind you.

Dealing with Grief and Loss

As you consider your losses, consider the following tips to help you work through your feelings without becoming immobilized by any one emotion.

- Permit yourself to experience your feelings. Face your loss; let yourself grieve, cry, and be sad. Don't try to ignore anger or punish yourself for feeling it. These emotions are a normal part of the grieving process. As long as they don't hang around too long, they can help you move on to a more comfortable state of mind. However, if severe depression and crying continue for more than two weeks, see a doctor.

- Find out what triggers your fears and emotions. What led up to your feeling? What do you need right now that you don't have? If you know you get depressed around certain times of the year, such as an anniversary date, plan to take special care of yourself during that time or plan a special treat for yourself. Avoid situations that create anxiety. This includes limiting the amount of time you spend around people who make you feel uncomfortable.

- Express your fears and feelings and then let them go. Repressing your feelings can be a form of denial or it can stem from fear of alienating friends and family. Repressed feelings can fester and grow. Bottling up anger, for example, can result in excessive irritability, bitterness, and quarreling. Repressed feelings can also come out in other destructive ways, such as not following your prescribed treatment. Some constructive ways of expressing your feelings include: talking with others, writing in a journal, crying, screaming in the shower, or pounding pillows.

- Search for meaning. Draw strength from your spiritual beliefs. Also, think about what positive things have occurred as a result of your fibromyalgia that might not have happened otherwise. For example you may have:

  – reassessed priorities
  – discovered inner strengths
  – developed new hobbies
  – discovered new talents
  – made new friends
  – increased your understanding of yourself
  – increased your understanding of God, a higher power, or spirituality
  – increased your understanding of others with disabilities.

- Seek professional help when needed. Often, just talking with an understanding person will be enough to help you through depression or grief. But if you are having trouble maintaining your daily activities, feel helpless or hopeless, or have thought of hurting yourself or others, seek professional help at once. See the end of this chapter for help on finding referrals.

Self-Talk

Self-talk is the "little voice in your head" you use to talk to and think about yourself. It colors your world view and shapes your expectations. When self-talk is healthy, the little voice is a cheering section urging you forward to achieve success. When it's unhealthy, self-talk holds you back.

Unhealthy self-talk arises from automatically responding to situations with the same erroneous thinking pattern. These errors in thinking include a tendency to overgeneralize, to see things in terms of right/wrong and good/bad, to "catastrophize," to place undue significance on only one aspect of an event, and to jump to conclusions. Your self-talk is unhealthy when you get stuck just thinking negative thoughts.

It isn't difficult to diagnose thinking errors if you watch for "red flags" in the way you talk to yourself. Look for red flags when you categorize people or yourself, or when you judge, label, or condemn. They should also arise with frequent use of words and phrases like *can't,*

won't, impossible, always, never, should, ought to, must, yes but, if only . . .
Here are some examples of unhealthy ways of thinking.

10 Unhealthy Ways to Think

1. *Seeing all or nothing:* You place people or situations in black and white categories, with no shades of gray. If your performance falls short of perfect, you see yourself as a total failure.

2. *Overgeneralizing:* You see a single unhealthy event as a never-ending pattern of defeat.

3. *Using mental filters:* You pick out a single unhealthy detail and dwell on it exclusively so that your vision of all reality becomes darkened, like the drop of ink that discolors the entire beaker of water.

4. *Disqualifying the healthy:* You reject healthy experiences by insisting they "don't count" for some reason or other. In this way you can maintain an unhealthy belief that is contradicted by your everyday experiences.

5. *Jumping to conclusions:* You make an unhealthy interpretation even though there are no definite facts that convincingly support your conclusion. Some examples:
   a. *Mind reading:* You arbitrarily conclude that someone is reacting negatively to you and don't bother to find out if that's true.
   b. *Fortune telling:* You anticipate that things will turn out badly, and you feel convinced that your prediction is an already-established fact.

6. *Magnifying or minimizing:* You exaggerate the importance of insignificant events (such as your goof-up or someone else's achievement), or you inappropriately shrink significant ones until they appear tiny (your own desirable qualities or the other fellow's imperfections). This is also called the "binocular trick."

7. *Basing facts on your emotions:* You assume that your unhealthy emotions necessarily reflect the way things really are: "I feel it, therefore it must be true."

8. *Using "should" statements:* You try to motivate yourself with *shoulds* and *shouldn'ts,* as if you had to be whipped and punished before you could be expected to do anything. ("I really should exercise. I shouldn't be so lazy.") "Musts" and "oughts" are also offenders. The emotional consequence is guilt. When you direct "should" statements toward others, you feel anger, frustration, and resentment.

9. *Labeling and mislabeling:* This is an extreme form of overgener-

alizing. Instead of describing your error, you attach a unhealthy label to yourself: "I'm a loser."

When someone else's behavior rubs you the wrong way, you attach an unhealthy label to him: "He's a real louse." Mislabeling involves describing an event with language that is highly colored and emotionally loaded. Example: Instead of saying someone drops off her children at day care every day, you might say she "abandons her children and lets strangers look after them."

10. *Personalizing:* You see yourself as the cause of some unhealthy external event which in fact you were not primarily responsible for.

Thought Stopping

Unhealthy self-talk can make the challenges presented by fibromyalgia seem like an uphill, unwinnable battle. Learning to change your self-talk from distorted to helpful is an important tool in reducing your stress and improving your mood. Here are some ways to do this.

Changing Unhealthy Self-Talk

Unhealthy: "I would like to exercise but I can't. I know if I did any exercise my fibromyalgia would act up. I am also too old to start exercising. I know I can't do it."

Healthy: "Starting an exercise program will give me a chance to get outdoors again. I could start slow and easy with a walk in the mall. If I get tired, I can sit down and look at store windows and rest for a while." Or: "Starting an exercise program will be a challenge, but I can take it slowly and it will give me a chance to . . . ."

Unhealthy: "My life will never be the same now that I have fibromyalgia. I will never be able to do anything that I like to do."

Healthy: "I'm still the same person I've always been. I can cope." Or: "I've changed since I was diagnosed with fibromyalgia but I'm still a person of worth. I still have a lot to give to people around me."

Unhealthy: "My friends never call me. People don't like being around me anymore."

Healthy: "My friends are just trying to be considerate and spare my energy. They are waiting on signals from me. I'll call today!" Or: "My friends are uncomfortable, at a loss, and don't know how to help me. I must ask them for what I need."

ON A PERSONAL NOTE

Redefining a Mother's Role
by Andrea Acker, Lilburn, GA

After struggling for seven months to cope with fibromyalgia, I felt guilty for not being able to do the things I used to do for my family. My role as a mother was threatened because I thought my kids no longer needed me. I decided I needed to change that role in order to adapt to our new situation. Maybe my kids don't need me as much anymore, but there's no sense in punishing them for growing up.

One afternoon, my son came to me asking advice about a problem he was having at school. I told him how I would handle it, and he seemed satisfied. Then it hit me: My kids do still need me, but now in a different way. I can offer them motherly guidance, using my head and my heart, rather than my body, to help them. I decided to no longer try to do for them what they are capable of doing for themselves. But children always need someone to listen.

Reprinted from Arthritis Today, November/October 1996.

GETTING SELF-TALK TO WORK FOR YOU

- Write down self-defeating thoughts.
- Do a "Reality Check." Ask:

    – Are there other ways of looking at this situation?
    – What am I afraid will occur?
    – How do I know that this will indeed happen?
    – What evidence do I have that this will happen?
    – Is there evidence that contradicts this conclusion?
    – What coping resources are available?
    – Have I only had failures in the past, or were there times I did okay?
    – There are times when I don't do as well as I would like, but other times I do, so what are the differences between those times?

- Change self-defeating thoughts to helpful self-talk.
- Mentally rehearse healthy self-talk.
- Practice healthy self-talk in real situations.
- Be patient—it takes time for new patterns of thinking to become automatic.

ACTIVITY: Keep a Thoughts Diary

Paying attention to your thoughts and feelings is the first step in gaining control of unpleasant emotions. But during times of emotional turmoil, your thoughts may be so fragmented and jumbled that it's hard to know exactly what they are. Writing in a journal or in a "Thoughts Diary" is an excellent way to explore your thoughts and feelings (see Sample Thoughts Diary on page 35). Because it's your private document, a diary can be a good "safety-valve" for dealing with emotions and stress.

A diary or journal can also help you catch yourself in unhealthy thinking, can serve as a reality check, and can help you process your feelings and thoughts. After you've been writing your thoughts down for a few weeks or months, look back at some of your earlier entries. You may find your perspective has changed. See Chapter 3 for more information on self-management.

Avoiding a Spiral into Depression

Reactions like anger, fear, and anxiety are normal parts of the grieving process. They are signals from the body and mind that all is not well and that it is time to mobilize your coping responses. When these emotions are processed by a healthy grieving person, they can provide an opportunity to grow and gain new insights. But if they are not dealt with appropriately, they can cause long-term depression. The goal is to process and listen to your feelings, and then release them.

How to Know if You're Depressed

Depression has become a catchall term. The word is sometimes used inappropriately to refer to brief feelings of sadness or dissatisfaction. Experiencing a few depressive symptoms every now and then is part of life. But true depression alters the way you view the world and yourself. It can be a vague unhappiness that lasts for several days. Or it can be long-lasting, interfering with your ability to take pleasure in life, disrupting sleep, and causing you to feel helpless and hopeless. Depression can also cover other emotions that are painful to face, like anger or guilt.

It can be hard to recognize depression when you're in the middle of it. Because it can come on gradually, depression can take hold of you before you realize what has happened. The chart of symptoms below will help you determine whether depression may be dragging you down as much as or more than your fibromyalgia.

Remember that fibromyalgia itself, as well as medications used to treat it, can cause some of the symptoms listed on this chart, particularly low energy and fatigue, changes in appetite and weight, and sleeping too much or too little. So these symptoms alone may not indicate depression. However, you should seek professional help if you have four or more additional symptoms that last for more than two weeks and are severe enough to disrupt your daily life. If you have suicidal thoughts, seek professional help immediately. Don't let your sad mood become a tragedy. Remember, even the most severe depression is treatable and temporary.

ACTIVITY   Depression—A self-test

Experiencing one or more of these depressive symptoms every now and then is a normal part of life. If a certain number of these symptoms have been bothering you for weeks or years, you may have a depressive disorder and should consult your doctor with this list in hand. See "Results" below.

Group 1:
Are you experiencing at least one of the following nearly every day?:
- apathy, or loss of interest in things you used to enjoy, including sex
- sadness, blues, or irritability

Group 2:
In addition, are you experiencing any of the following?:
- feeling slowed down or restless
- feeling worthless or guilty
- changes in appetite or weight (a loss or gain of either)
- thoughts of death or suicide (not necessarily attempts at suicide)*
- problems concentrating, thinking, remembering, or making decisions
- trouble falling asleep or sleeping too much
- loss of energy, feeling tired all the time

Group 3:
And what about the following symptoms? These are not used to diagnose depressive disorders, but often occur with them.
- headaches**
- other aches and pains **
- digestive problems**

- sexual problems**
- feeling pessimistic or hopeless
- being anxious or worried
- low self-esteem

Results:

If you have several symptoms, talk to your physician. You may be in a major depressive episode if you are experiencing at least one of the symptoms in Group 1 and at least four of the symptoms in Group 2 nearly every day for at least two weeks.

You may have chronic depression if you experience at least one of the symptoms in Group 1 and at least two of the symptoms in Group 2 nearly every day for at least two years.

*Suicide attempts or thoughts are never a part of healthy thought patterns and should never be written off as the blues. If you have these thoughts, seek professional help.

**These are potential indications of depression only if not caused by another disease.

Reprinted from *Arthritis Today*, January/February 1996.

RISK FACTORS OF DEPRESSION

YOU ARE AT RISK FOR DEPRESSION IF:

- You have had a prior depressive episode.
- Your first depressive episode occurred before you were age 40.
- You have a medical condition.
- You have just given birth.
- You have very little or no social support.
- You have undergone a stressful life event, either positive or negative.
- You abuse alcohol or drugs.
- You have a family history of depressive disorders.
- You received only partial relief from an earlier episode of depression.

*Reprinted from **Arthritis Today**, January/February 1996.*

Seeking Professional Help

If you determine that you are depressed, help is available. Seeing a mental-health professional once carried a stigma, but no longer. It's now widely recognized that seeing a therapist for help in sorting out your feelings is no different from seeing a dentist for a cavity or a doctor for the flu. A psychiatrist or psychologist can help you work through your thoughts and emotions by providing an objective, listening ear and offering insight into what you may be feeling or thinking.

Even if you're not significantly depressed, you can still benefit greatly from therapy. Dealing with the pain, fatigue, and lifestyle changes imposed by fibromyalgia can be an enormous psychological challenge. Mental or emotional patterns that caused minor trouble earlier may now cause major problems. Relationships that functioned satisfactorily without the stress of illness may now call for restructuring and greatly improved communication skills. Or, you may simply need a safe place to discuss your feelings. For any of these reasons, therapy might prove extremely valuable. You are worth getting the help you need or simply want.

Once you have made the decision to seek help from a therapist, how do you go about finding a qualified therapist in your area? Start by getting a list of therapists your insurance company will cover. Take this list with you as you ask around for references. Your own physician may have some good suggestions. A trustworthy friend or relative who has been pleased with the services of a mental-health practitioner may be able to recommend someone. Another way to find a qualified therapist is to call a reputable hospital or mental-health agency in your area.

It is well worth shopping around to find a qualified person with whom you can feel comfortable. Today, any number of people call themselves therapists although they have no licenses or training. There is nothing illegal about this, and some of them may be good at what they do. But your best bet is to make sure that the person you choose has appropriate education and training and belongs to the recognized professional organization for his or her license (e.g., the National Association of Social Workers). Often, such an organization will have its own referral telephone line, which will be listed in the Yellow Pages. The person you find may be a board-certified psychiatrist (MD); licensed clinical psychologist (PhD); licensed clinical social worker (MSW/LCSW); or licensed marriage, family, and child counselor (MFCC). Therapists who are not medical doctors, and who thus cannot prescribe drugs, may refer you for psychiatric consultation to evaluate your need for medication. See Chapter 4 for more information about different types of doctors and therapists.

Once you have obtained some names, don't hesitate to interview a prospective therapist on the phone. Ask questions about qualifications, training, and specific areas of expertise. Ask how much experience the doctor or therapist has had in treating depression. Some therapists have special knowledge about this illness, and it is perfectly appropriate to ask. You have a right to this information, and a competent professional will not be offended by your questions. Some therapists are willing to meet with you for an initial session without charge, so that you can make an in-person evaluation.

If your insurance doesn't cover therapy, don't let that stop you from seeking the help you need. Community mental-health agencies usually use a sliding-fee scale, based on the patient's income, family size, and other considerations. Some private practitioners significantly lower their fees on a financial-need basis. Good, affordable help is available.

WHERE TO FIND HELP

The following organizations offer general information on depressive disorders, mental illness, and how to find a therapist. Some also have a referral service to help you find a credentialed therapist in your area.

American Association for Marriage and Family Therapy, 1133 15th St., NW, Suite 300, Washington, DC 20005; 800/374-2638.

American Psychiatric Association, Department AT, 1400 K St., NW, Washington, DC 20002; 202/682-6220.

American Psychological Association, 750 First St., NE, Washington, DC 20002; 800/374-3120.

Depression Awareness, Recognition and Treatment (D/ART), a program of the National Institute of Mental Health, 5600 Fischers La., Room 10-85, Rockville, MD 20857; 800/421-4211.

National Alliance for the Mentally Ill, 200 N. Blebe Rd., Suite 1015, Arlington, VA 22203-3754; 800/950-6264.

National Association of Social Workers, 750 First St., NE, Suite 700, Washington, DC 20002; 202/408-8600.

National Depressive and Manic Depressive Association, 730 N. Franklin, Suite 501, Chicago, IL 60610; 800/82N-DMDA or 800/826-3632.

National Foundation for Depressive Illness, P.O. Box 2257, New York, NY 10116; 800/248-4344.

National Mental Health Association, 1021 Prince St., Alexandria, VA 22314-2971; 800/969-6642.

*Reprinted from **Arthritis Today**, January/February 1996.*

PART FOUR
Living Well with Fibromyalgia

In this section, self-help is taken to the next step, to proactively building your health to prevent problems. That means adopting a "wellness lifestyle."

A wellness lifestyle is one in which you are committed to nourishing your body and mind. It includes attitudes and behaviors that help you achieve the highest possible physical, mental, and spiritual well-being.

The following chapters are devoted to exercise, diet, and positive communication, all necessary keys to living well.

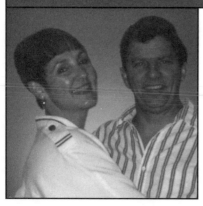

Lisa Pulyer and her husband

Exercising Your Right to a Better Life with Fibromyalgia
by Lisa Pulyer
Grants Pass, OR

In 1990, after suffering unexplained pain and fatigue for the previous two years, I finally found a very sharp young rheumatologist who diagnosed my illness as fibromyalgia. My doctor warned me that the medications she would prescribe would do little to relieve the severe symptoms of fibromyalgia, but they would take the edge off the pain and help me sleep. She also told me that mild exercise would be my best defense by keeping my muscles, tendons, and ligaments as strong and flexible as possible. Instead, I used my pain and fatigue as an excuse not to exercise. My illness was beginning to control my life. Not only did it invade every aspect of my life, it also caused my self-esteem to plummet. I became a shadow of my pre-fibromyalgia self.

In 1993, when I realized I had gone from 118 pounds to 138 pounds in less than one year and I was staring my fortieth birthday in the face, I panicked. Not only did I feel rotten physically and mentally, I also looked rotten. I started to exercise slowly, 20 minutes on a stationary bicycle once or twice a week. That wasn't enough to make much of a difference in my weight, but I quickly began to feel the benefits of an increase in energy and a decrease in pain severity. I started to take back some control of my life. I was doing something to control my illness, not let my illness control me.

The more I exercised, the better I felt. I started to exercise three to four days a week. I developed a weight-training program that I could tolerate as well as doing 15 miles per workout on the bike. The weight slowly started to come off, and I began to work out five days a week. I felt and looked better all the time. Before, I used my pain as an excuse not to exercise. Now, the more pain I'm in, the more important exercising has become to me.

I still suffer daily pain and a certain amount of fatigue, and I know I have limitations. Now, however, instead of allowing my flares to send me to bed, I exercise through them if at all possible, and the pain does not last as long as it did when I would just lie in bed.

I now know that I will have to exercise, in some fashion, for the rest of my life in order to be able to live with fibromyalgia. Too bad that vanity was the prevailing force behind my exercising. I could have spared myself three years of disability!

CHAPTER TEN

Exercising

Why Exercise?

Some kind of exercise is good for almost everyone, but it can be especially helpful for people with fibromyalgia. Two principles of treatment for fibromyalgia are to increase cardiovascular (aerobic) fitness and to stretch and mobilize tight, sore muscles and strengthen them. Research has shown it is possible to improve general health and fitness through exercise without increasing fibromyalgia symptoms.

If the idea of starting an exercise program intimidates you, remember that exercise can be beneficial. If you feel you can't maintain a regular, strenuous workout at first, do whatever you can. As you become stronger and your endurance increases, you may be able to increase your workout.

Exercise is beneficial for people with fibromyalgia in a number of ways. It can:

- keep your body from becoming too stiff
- keep your muscles strong
- keep bone and cartilage tissue strong and healthy
- improve your ability to do daily activities
- give you more energy
- help you sleep better
- control your weight
- make your heart stronger and improve your cardiovascular health
- provide an outlet for stress and tension
- decrease depression and anxiety
- release endorphins, your body's natural pain relievers
- improve your self-esteem and provide a sense of well-being.

What If I Don't Exercise?

If your body hurts or you're tired, you may not feel like exercising. However, as one old saying goes "If you don't use it, you lose it." Healthy people who are given bed rest rapidly decondition, suffering decreasing heart muscle, reduced blood volume, atrophied muscles, decreased bone density, and light-headedness upon getting out of bed.

As the diagram here shows, going without exercise can result in a cycle of deconditioning that leads to further pain. People in pain tend to guard painful parts and reduce their activities. This creates stiffness and increased muscle tension, leading to even more pain. Add to this the effects of a poor night's sleep. Who has the energy to move?

Inactivity causes deconditioning: Your muscles become smaller and weaker and are less able to support and protect you. You have less stamina and get tired more easily. Daily activities are more difficult to do. This loss in function and independence can lead to depression, anger, and lowered self-esteem, which in turn result in stress, which creates muscle tension, leading to more pain, and so on through the cycle. Exercise is one of the prime weapons used to break this cycle. Research has shown that participating in a regular exercise program is a great way to feel better and move more comfortably with less pain.

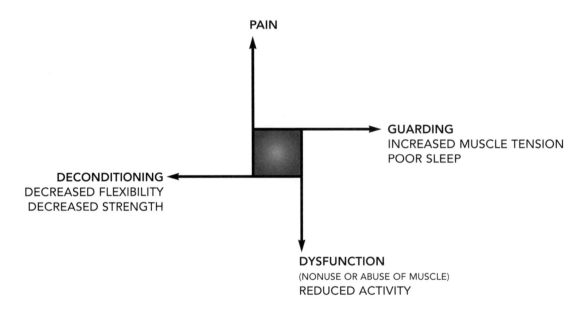

Pain, Guarding, Dysfunction and Deconditioning

Three Essential Parts of an Exercise Program

Everyone, including people with fibromyalgia, benefits from a balanced exercise program including different types of exercise: warm-up, endurance (aerobics), and cool-down.

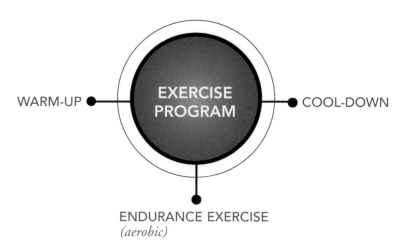

WARM-UP ● **EXERCISE PROGRAM** ● COOL-DOWN

ENDURANCE EXERCISE
(aerobic)

Three Parts of an Exercise Program

Warm-up

Be sure to warm up with some easy marching, walking, or arm swings before exercising. This includes range-of-motion, stretching, and some strengthening exercises. Warm-up exercises safely prepare your heart and lungs for endurance and help maintain or increase flexibility and muscle strength. For some people with severe physical limitations, this may be the only type of exercise they can do initially.

Endurance Exercises

Also called aerobic exercises, these exercises use the large muscles of the body and increase the heart rate. They are important for cardiovascular fitness, weight control, and lessening of fatigue. They include swimming, walking, and bicycling. Work into these activities gradually.

Cool-down

A cool-down period is necessary to let your body lose some of the heat it has generated while exercising. This will help relax your body, return your heart rate to normal, and avoid sore muscles. To cool down, your chosen aerobic exercise should be done in slow motion for three to five minutes, followed by a few flexibility and stretching exercises.

A Look at Different Types of Exercise

To create your fitness program, you should combine some type of flexibility and muscle-strengthening exercises with endurance exercises. You may not be able to do all of these every day. Let the way you're feeling on a particular day be your guide.

Range-of-Motion (Flexibility/Stretching) Exercises

Range-of-motion (ROM) exercises are beneficial because they reduce stiffness and help keep your muscles and joints flexible. The range of motion is the full range in which your joints can be moved in certain directions. A physical therapist can teach you appropriate range-of-motion exercises.

You should try to move your joints through their full range of motion every day. Daily activities such as housework, climbing stairs, dressing, bathing, cooking, lifting, or bending do not dependably move your joints through their full range of motion and should not replace range-of-motion exercises prescribed by your doctor or therapist.

Some ROM exercises can be used to stretch or elongate the ligaments and muscles around the joint. This stretching helps maintain or improve the flexibility of these tissues. Stretching is also used to reduce muscle tension. A sustained, gentle, nonpainful stretch to a tight muscle will assist in relaxing that muscle, thereby improving flexibility and reducing pain.

Strengthening Exercises

These exercises are beneficial because they help maintain or increase muscle strength. Strong muscles help keep your body conditioned and better able to withstand the painful effects of fibromyalgia. Two common strengthening exercises are isometric and isotonic exercises.

Isometric Exercises

In these exercises, you tighten your muscles but don't move your joints. This helps build the muscles around your joints. Examples of isometric exercises are quadriceps sets, in which you tighten the large muscle on the front of your thigh muscles, or gluteal sets, in which you tighten the muscles in your buttocks.

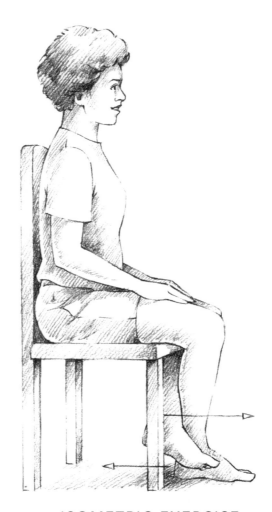

ISOMETRIC EXERCISE
This exercise strengthens the muscles that bend and straighten your knee. Sit in a straight-backed chair and cross your ankles. Your legs can be almost straight, or you can bend your knees as much as you like. Push forward with your back leg and press backward with your front leg. Exert pressure evenly so that your legs do not move. Hold and count out loud for 10 seconds. Relax. Change leg positions.

Isotonic Exercises

In these exercises, you move your joints to strengthen your muscles. For example, straightening your knee while sitting in a chair is an isotonic exercise that helps strengthen your thigh muscle. Isotonic exercises include range-of-motion exercises, but they become strengthening exercises when you increase the speed at which they are done, increase the repetition of exercises that are done, or add weight to the exercise being done (initially one to two pounds).

Water exercises can help strengthen muscles because water gives resistance as well as assistance to movements. Changing the position in which you do exercises also can help strengthen muscles. For example, you encounter more resistance when you raise your arms from a sitting position than when you raise your arms from a lying-down position.

Strengthening exercises must be carefully designed for people with fibromyalgia. Knowing which muscle needs to be strengthened and how to perform the exercise without overstressing your joints and muscles are key elements in a successful program.

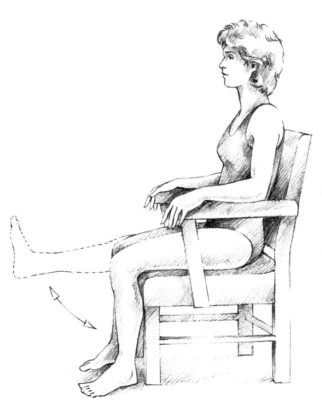

ISOTONIC EXERCISE
This exercise strengthens your thigh muscles. Sit in a chair with both feet on the floor and spread slightly apart. Raise one foot until your leg is as straight as you can make it. Hold and count out loud for five seconds. Gently lower your foot to the floor. Relax. Repeat with your other leg.

Sample Exercises

Here are some sample range-of-motion and strengthening exercises that you can use in either a warm-up or a cool-down. Select the exercises that are best for you depending upon which areas are painful.

Note: These exercises have been excerpted from the Arthritis Foundation's PACE® Exercise Program Instructor's Manual, © Arthritis Foundation, 1993.

NECK EXERCISES

Purpose: Increase neck movement. Relax tense neck and shoulder muscles. Improve posture.

Precautions: Do slowly and smoothly. If you feel dizzy, stop the exercise. If you have had neck problems, check with your doctor before doing these exercises.

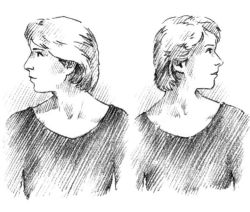

2 HEAD TURNS (ROTATION)
Turn your head to look over your shoulder. Hold three seconds. Return to the center and then turn to look over your other shoulder. Hold three seconds. Repeat.

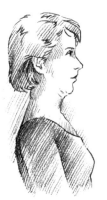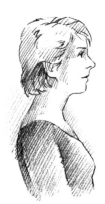

1 CHIN TUCKS
Pull your chin back as if to make a double chin. Keep your head straight – don't look down. Hold three seconds. Then raise your neck straight up as if someone was pulling straight up on your hair.

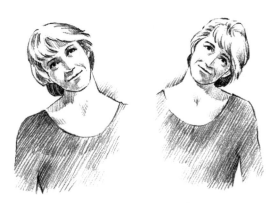

3 HEAD TILTS
Focus on an object in front of you. Tilt your head sideways toward your right shoulder. Hold three seconds. Return to the center and tilt toward your left shoulder. Hold three seconds. Do not twist you head but continue to look forward. Do not raise your shoulder toward your ear.

SHOULDER GIRDLE EXERCISES

Purpose: Increase mobility of the shoulder girdle (the bony structure that supports the upper limbs). Strengthen muscles that raise shoulders. Relax tense neck and shoulder muscles.

Precautions: If the exercise increases pain, stop and consult with your physician.

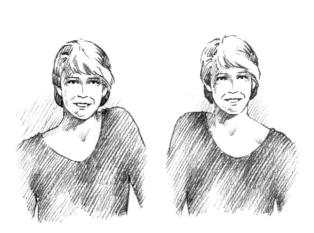

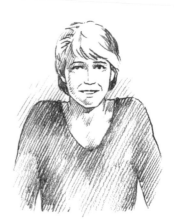

4 SHOULDER SHRUGS (ELEVATION)
A) **Raise one shoulder, lower it. Then raise the other shoulder. Be sure the first shoulder is completely relaxed and lowered before raising the other.**

B) **Raise both shoulders up toward the ears. Hold three seconds. Relax. Concentrate on completely relaxing shoulders as they come down. Do not tilt the head or body in either direction. Do not hunch the shoulders forward or pinch the shoulder blades together.**

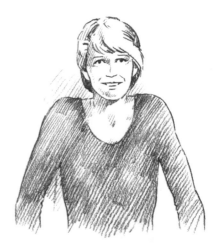

5 SHOULDER CIRCLES
Lift both shoulders up, move them forward, then down and back in a circling motion. Then lift both shoulders up, move them backward, then down and forward in a circling motion.

ARM EXERCISES (for shoulders and elbows)

Purpose: Increase shoulder and/or elbow motion. Strengthen shoulder and/or elbow muscles. Relax tense neck and shoulder muscles. Improve posture.

Precautions: If you have had shoulder or elbow surgery, check with your surgeon before doing these exercises. These exercises are also not advisable for people with significant shoulder joint damage, such as unstable joints and partial or total cuff tears.

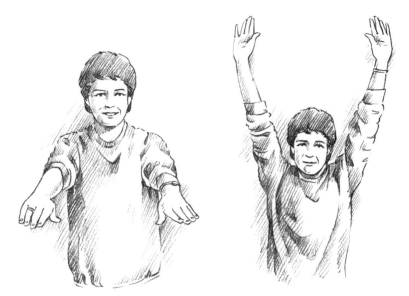

6 FORWARD ARM REACH (FLEXION)
Raise one or both arms forward and upward as high as possible. Return to your starting position.

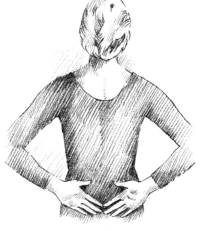

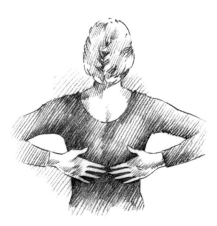

7 SELF BACK RUB
(INTERNAL ROTATION)
While sitting, slide a few inches forward from the back of the chair. Try to sit up straight and not round your shoulders. Place the back of your hands on your lower back. Slowly move them upward until you feel a stretch in your shoulders. Hold three seconds, then slide your hands back down. You can use one hand to help the other. Move within the limits of your pain. Do not force.

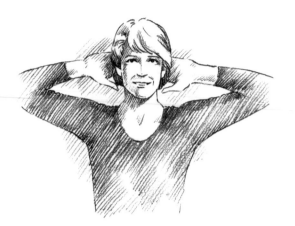
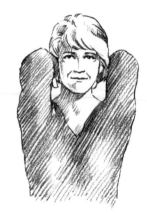

8 SHOULDER ROTATOR
Sit or stand as straight as possible. Reach up and place your
hands on the back of your head. (If you cannot reach your head,
place your arms in a "muscle man" position with elbows bent
in a right angle and upper arm at shoulder level.) Take a deep
breath in. As you breathe out, bring your elbows together.
Slowly move your elbows apart as you breathe in.

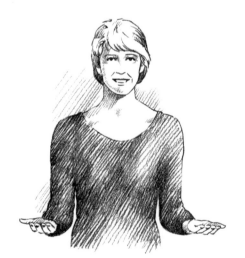
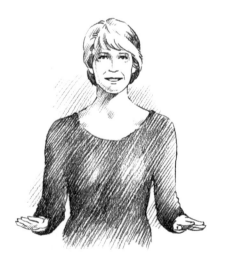

9 DOOR OPENER (PRONATION AND SUPINATION)
Bend your elbows and hold them into your sides.
Your forearms should be parallel to the floor. Slowly turn
your forearms and palms to face the ceiling. Hold three
seconds and then turn them toward the floor.

WRIST EXERCISES

Purpose: Increase wrist motion. Strengthen wrist muscles.

Precaution: If you have had wrist or elbow surgery, check with your doctor before doing this exercise. Stop if you feel any numbness or tingling.

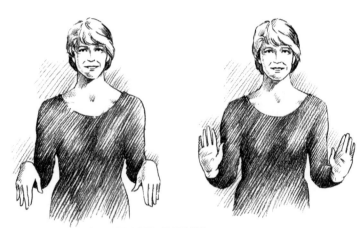

10 WRIST BEND (EXTENSION)

If sitting, rest hands and forearms on thighs, table or arms of the chair. If standing, bend your elbows and hold hands in front of you, palms down. Lift up palms and fingers, keeping forearms flat. Hold three seconds. Relax.

FINGER EXERCISES

Purpose: Increase finger motion. Increase ability to hold objects.

Precautions: If the exercise increases pain, stop and consult with your physician.

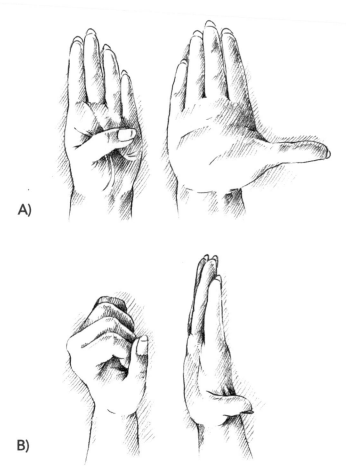

A)

B)

11 THUMB BEND AND FINGER CURL
(THUMB AND FINGER FLEXION/EXTENSION)
A)With hands open and fingers relaxed, reach your thumb across your palm and try to touch the base of the little finger. Hold three seconds. Stretch thumb back out to the other side as far as possible. B)Then make a loose fist by curling all your fingers into your palm. Keep your thumb out. Hold for three seconds. Then stretch out your fingers to straighten them.

TRUNK EXERCISES

Purpose: Increase trunk flexibility. Stretch and strengthen back and abdominal muscles.

Precautions: If you have osteoporosis, back compression fracture, previous back surgery or a hip replacement, check with your doctor before doing these exercises. Do not bend your body forward or backward unless specifically told to do so. Move slowly and immediately stop any exercise that causes you any back or neck pain.

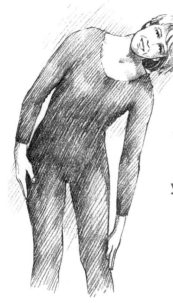

12 SIDE BENDS
While standing, keep weight evenly on both hips. Lean toward the right and reach your fingers toward the floor. Hold three seconds. Return to center and repeat exercise toward the left. Do not lean forward or backward and don't twist.

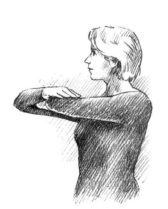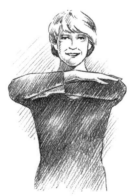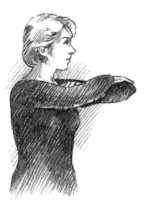

13 TRUNK TWIST (ROTATION)
Place your hands on your hips, straight out to the side, crossed over your chest or on opposite elbows. Twist your body around to look over your right shoulder. Hold three seconds. Return to the center and then twist to the left. Be sure you are twisting at the waist and not at your neck or hips. NOTE: You can vary the exercise by holding a ball in front of or next to your body.

LOWER BODY EXERCISES

Position: Stand upright with shoulders back, arms at side and stomach pulled in. Relax knees to avoid locked-knee position.

Precautions: Check with your surgeon before doing the following exercise if you have had hip, knee, ankle, foot or toe surgery. Do not do this exercise if you have pain in the balls of your feet.

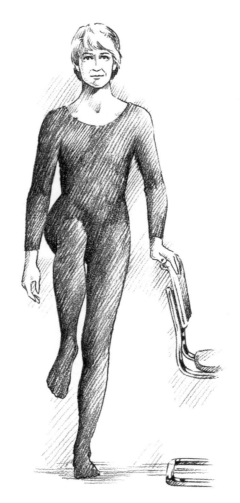

14 MARCH
(HIP/KNEE FLEXION)
Stand sideways to a chair and lightly
hold onto the back. If you feel
unsteady, hold onto two chairs or
face the back of the chair. Alternate
lifting your legs up and down as if
you were marching in place. Gradually
try to lift higher and/or faster.

Precautions: If you have had a hip replacement, talk to your surgeon before doing the following exercise.

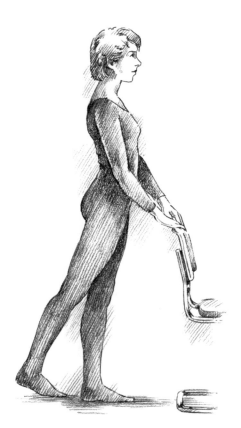

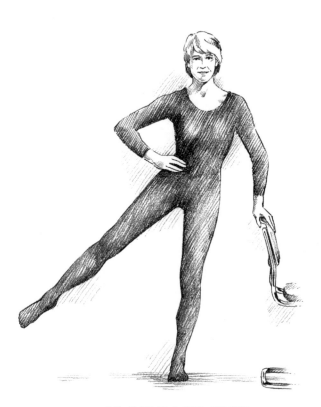

15 BACK KICK
(HIP EXTENSION)

Stand straight on one leg and lift your other leg behind you. Hold three seconds. Try to keep your leg straight as you move it backward. Motion should only occur in hip (not waist). Do not lean forward – keep your upper body straight. NOTE: You can add resistance by using a large rubber exercise band around ankles.

16 SIDE LEG KICK
(HIP ABDUCTION/ADDUCTION)

Stand near a chair, holding it for support. Stand on one leg and lift the other leg out to side. Hold three seconds and return your leg to the floor. Only move your leg at the top – don't lean toward the chair. Alternate legs.

Precautions: Check with your surgeon before doing the following exercises if you have had a hip replacement. Keep the knee bent in the weight-bearing leg. Don't rotate your upper body–keep your chest and shoulders facing forward.

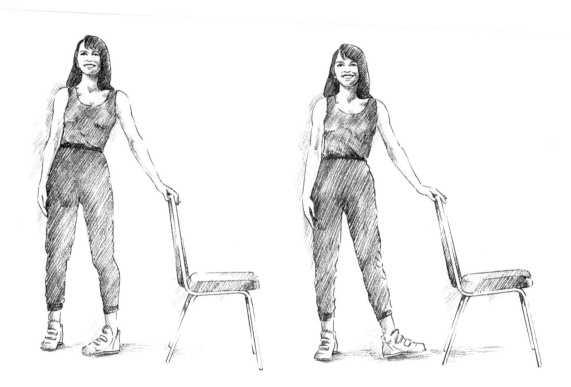

17 HIP TURNS (HIP INTERNAL/EXTERNAL ROTATION)
Stand with your legs slightly apart, weight on one leg and the heel of your other leg lightly touching the floor. Rotate your whole leg from the hip so that toes and knee point in and then out. Don't rotate your body – keep your chest and shoulders facing forward.
NOTE: If you have difficulty putting weight on one leg, you can also do this exercise by sitting at the edge of the chair with your legs extended straight in front and with your heels resting on the floor.

Precautions: Check with your surgeon before doing the following exercises if you have had a hip replacement. Don't rotate your upper body–keep your chest and shoulders facing forward.

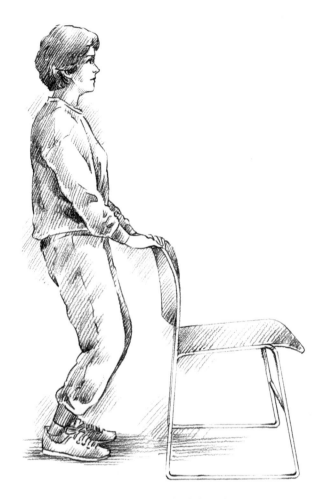

18 SKIER'S SQUAT
(QUADRICEPS STRENGTHENER)
Stand behind a chair with your hands lightly resting on top of the chair for support. Keep your feet flat on the floor. Slowly bend your knees to lower your body a few inches. Hold to the count of three to six and then slowly return to an upright position. Keep your back straight.

Precautions: Do not do the following exercise if you have had ankle or foot surgery. Stop if you experience calf pain or cramping.

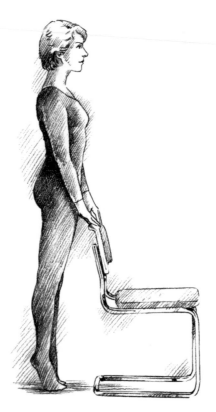

19 TIPTOE
(DORSI/PLANTARFLEXION)
Face the back of the chair and rest your
hands on it. Rise up and stand on your toes.
Hold three seconds then return to the flat
position. Try to keep your knees straight.
Now stand on your heels, raising your toes
and front part of your foot off the ground.
NOTE: You can do this one foot at a time.

Precautions: If you have had recent ankle surgery, check with your surgeon before doing the following exercise.

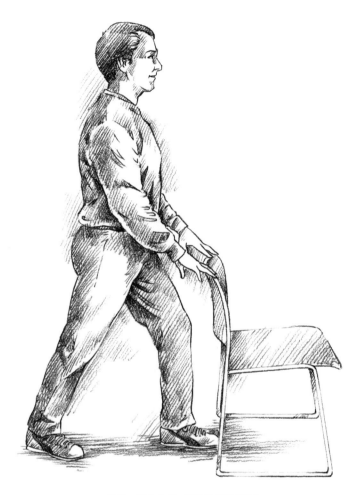

20 CALF STRETCH
(GASTROC-SOLEUS STRETCH)
Hold lightly to the back of a chair. Bend the knee
of the leg you are not stretching so it almost touches
the chair. Put the leg to be stretched behind you,
keeping both feet flat on the floor. Lean forward,
keeping your back knee straight.

Precautions: Stop if the following exercise increases your back pain.

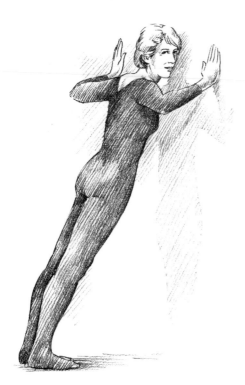

21 CHEST STRETCH
(HIP EXTENSION AND PECTORALIS STRETCH)
Stand about two to three feet away from a wall and place your hands or forearms on the wall at shoulder height. Lean forward, leading with your hips. Keep your knees straight and your head back. Hold this shoulder stretch position for five to 10 seconds. Push away. To feel more stretch, place your hands farther apart.

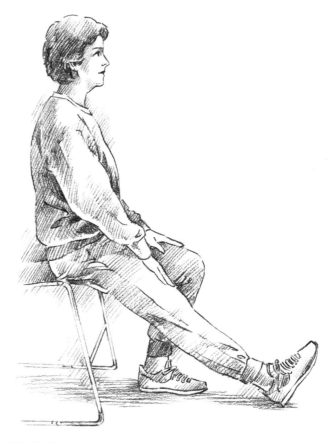

22 THIGH FIRMER AND KNEE STRETCH
Sit on the edge of a chair or lie on your back with your legs stretched out in front and your heels resting on the floor. Tighten the muscle that runs across the front of the knee by pulling your toes toward your head. Push the back of the knee down toward the floor so you also feel a stretch at the back of your knee and ankle. For a greater stretch, put your heel on a footstool and lean forward as you pull your toes toward your head.

Endurance Exercises

Endurance exercises (also called aerobic exercises) are beneficial because they strengthen your heart and make your lungs more efficient. They lessen fatigue by giving you more stamina so you can work longer without tiring as quickly. Endurance exercises also help you sleep better, control your weight, and lift your spirits.

Just about any exercise that uses the large muscles of the body in a continuous, rhythmic activity can be an endurance exercise, depending upon the person doing the exercise. For some, walking will increase fitness, while athletes must exercise vigorously to achieve an improvement in aerobic fitness. The signs that you are exercising at conditioning level are:

- increased heart rate
- increased breathing
- feeling warmer and/or sweating.

Some of the most beneficial endurance exercises for people with fibromyalgia are walking, water exercise, and using a stationary bicycle.

Walking

Walking requires no special skills and is inexpensive. However, you will need a good pair of supportive walking shoes. You can walk almost anytime and anywhere. Also, walking can be easily measured in terms of number of blocks or length of time, so it's easy to monitor your progress.

Water Exercise

Swimming and exercising in warm water are especially good for stiff, sore muscles. Warm water helps relax your muscles and decrease pain. The water should be between 83 and 87 degrees. Water helps support your body while you move your joints through their range of motion. With the water holding you up, there is less stress on your hips, knees, and spine. You can do warm-water exercises while standing in shoulder- or chest-height water or while sitting in shallow water. In deeper water, use an inflatable tube or flotation vest or belt to keep you afloat while you exercise.

Bicycling

Bicycling, especially on an indoor stationary bicycle, is a good way to improve your fitness without putting too much stress on your hips, knees, and feet. Some stationary bicycles have the capacity to exercise your upper body as well. Adjust the seat height so that your knee straightens when the pedal is at the lowest point. When you begin, do not pedal faster than 15 to 20 miles per hour, or 60 revolutions per minute. Add resistance only after you have warmed up for five minutes. Don't add so much resistance that you have trouble pedaling. If the cycling aggravates your pain, discuss this with your physician.

get FIT!

In planning and monitoring your endurance exercises, remember the "FIT" rule:

F **FREQUENCY** (NUMBER OF SESSIONS PER DAY PER WEEK):
If you are exercising less than five minutes each time, then eventually you should try to exercise several times each day. If you exercise five to 10 minutes at a time, then exercise twice a day. If you can exercise for more than 10 minutes at a time, then exercise once a day three to four times a week.

I **INTENSITY** (LEVEL OF DIFFICULTY):
The strenuousness of your workout will depend on your level of fitness, health, age and the activity of your fibromyalgia at a given time. But regardless, "going for the burn" is an outdated notion. It's not certain that the harder you work, the more benefit you'll reap. Exercise at no more than a moderate level. You should be able to talk as you exercise.

T **TIME** (LENGTH OF EACH SESSION):
Start with as little as one minute and gradually work up to 20 to 30 minutes of brisk exercise. This may take months to do. You can also accumulate 30 minutes of daily exercise by adding together three 10-minute sessions.

The goal of aerobic activity should be to work within your target heart rate range for a total of 30 minutes, at least three times a week whenever possible. Within these parameters, you should be able to steadily increase your fitness level. The following section will give you some guidelines to help you determine whether you're working too hard or not hard enough.

Understanding Perceived Exertion

When you are unsure of your pulse rate, try rating how hard you are working on a scale of zero to 10. Zero is equivalent to lying down and doing nothing. Ten is equal to working as hard as possible–very hard work that you could not do longer than seconds to minutes. A good level to aim for is between three and five, or moderate to strong exertion.

PERCEIVED EXERTION SCALE

0	Nothing at all
.5	Very, very weak
1	Very weak
2	Weak
3	Moderate
4	Somewhat strong
5	Strong
6	
7	Very strong
8	
9	
10	Very, very strong

Finding Your Target Heart Rate

Find the target heart rate for your age group in the following chart, and use it as a guide. You don't want your heart rate to be faster during peak exercise. If it is over the suggested heart rate at the time you count, slow the exercise. When you work out at this heart rate on a regular basis, your endurance and conditioning will improve.

You can measure your heart rate in beats per minute by counting your pulse for six seconds and adding a zero to that number (or by counting for 10 seconds and multiplying that number by six). For instance, if you count 20 beats in a 10-second period, your heart rate is six times 20, or 120 beats.

If you are a beginning exerciser, keep your heart rate at the low end of the range. Consider the upper number a "not to exceed" heart rate. To find your wrist pulse, hold your arm with your palm up, facing you. Bend your hand slightly away from you. Place the tips of your index and middle fingers of your other hand on the center of your wrist, slightly above the bend at your wrist. Slide your fingertips toward the outside of your wrist (the thumb side) and down over two tendons and into a soft depression between the tendons and the bone that runs along the thumb side of your wrist. Apply gentle pressure in that depression. Be sensitive to the pulsation there; it may take a little time to learn to feel your wrist pulse. It may be easier to find your pulse on one wrist than the other, so experiment to find which is easier for you.

Some people find it easier to feel their carotid pulse, located in the neck. To do this, put the tips of your index and middle fingers behind your earlobe and then slide them straight down and below your jawline. Apply gentle pressure; don't squeeze your neck between your thumb and fingers.

Don't stop your workout entirely as you take your pulse—it's important to keep your blood circulating. If possible, continue walking, cycling, or marching in place as you count. During water exercise, use a six-second heart rate, and your target heart rate will be the land heart rate minus 17.

THE TALK TEST

When you are exercising, you should be able to talk easily and not be out of breath. If you are exercising so hard that you can't talk normally, you may need to slow down.

RECOMMENDED HEART RATE RANGES

AGE	HEART RATE RANGE (60% - 75% of Age Predicted Maximum Heart Rate)	10-SECOND COUNT
20	120 – 150	20 – 25
25	117 – 146	19 – 24
30	114 – 143	19 – 24
35	111 – 139	18 – 23
40	108 – 135	18 – 23
45	105 – 131	17 – 22
50	102 – 128	17 – 21
55	99 – 124	16 – 21
60	96 – 120	16 – 20
65	93 – 116	15 – 19
70	90 – 113	15 – 19
75	87 – 109	14 – 18
80	84 – 105	14 – 18
85	81 – 101	13 – 17
90	78 – 98	13 – 16

How to Start Your Exercise Program

There are several different types of health professionals who can help you plan a total fitness program that will take into account your condition and your abilities. They can design a realistic fitness program that meets your specific needs.

- Start by asking your doctor for recommendations. He or she may recommend a regimen or may refer you to another health professional.
- Physical therapists can show you special exercises to help keep your bones and muscles strong and to increase your endurance.
- Occupational therapists can explain how to do exercises for your hands and can show you how to do your daily activities in ways that will help avoid fatigue and decrease stress on your body.
- Other professionals who can assist you are physiatrists, American College of Sports Medicine (ACSM) certified health and fitness instructors, personal trainers, and exercise physiologists.

Contact your doctor, local hospital-sponsored fitness facility, health clinic, or Arthritis Foundation chapter to learn about other exercise resources.

The toughest part of exercise, by far, is just getting started. But the effort you put into starting and maintaining a regular exercise program will come back to you a thousandfold in terms of better health, less pain, better sleep, and improved mental outlook. Once you've begun to enjoy the benefits of exercise, it will be easier to stick with it. Your body will start to feel more conditioned and you'll probably start to look forward to your workouts.

Stay Motivated

If you find it difficult to keep yourself motivated, consider these approaches:

- Set a regular time or times during the day to exercise. Write it on your calendar to remind yourself. Refer to the "Goal Setting and Contracting" section of Chapter 3. Use the contract form in Chapter 3 to set a realistic exercise goal you can achieve–write down what you plan to do and when you plan to do it. Have someone else sign the contract to help keep you motivated. Linking the time to something else makes it easier to make exercise a habit: for example, before your morning shower, before lunch, or after reading the newspaper.

- Stay in the habit by doing at least some exercise every day. On those days when you aren't motivated, it is especially important to make some effort, because interrupting the routine can not only decrease the benefits you get from exercise, it can quickly lead to abandoning the program altogether.

Monitor Your Progress

Before you get too far into a fitness program, it's a good idea to get a baseline fitness measurement, by which you can set goals and objectively evaluate your future progress. You can do this yourself by:

- doing a distance test. See how far you can walk, bicycle, or swim comfortably by measuring the distance on a marked running track, using the odometer on your car to measure street distance, using the bicycle odometer, or counting blocks or pool laps. Then measure how much more distance you can cover over time.
- doing a time test. Measure how long it took you to cover a certain distance, number of blocks, or pool lengths. Over time try to cover the same course in less time.
- measuring your heart rate or your perceived exertion rate and aiming to lower your rates over time.

Tips for Safe Exercise

Before Exercise

- Consult your physician or physical therapist before you begin a new fitness program.
- Warm up and slowly increase intensity before vigorous endurance-type exercise to help prevent injuries.
- Wear comfortable clothes and shoes. Your clothes should be loose and in layers so you can adapt to changes in temperature and activity. Your shoes should provide good support, and the soles should be made from nonslip, shock-absorbent material. Shock-absorbent insoles also can make your exercise more comfortable.

During Exercise

- Exercise at a comfortable, steady pace, and don't work so hard that you are out of breath (see the Talk Test in this chapter). Give your muscles time to relax between each repetition. For increased range of motion and flexibility, it is better to do each exercise slowly and completely rather than to do many repetitions at a fast pace.

- Remind yourself to breathe while you're working out—people often hold their breath during exercise without realizing it. When possible, exhale upon exertion and inhale during the release. Counting out loud during the exercise will help you breathe regularly. Don't try to breathe too deeply; just keep up your normal rate.

- Don't do too much too fast. Building endurance should be a gradual process spread out over several weeks or months. You can gradually increase the number of repetitions and times as you get into shape.

- Listen to your body. You may need to tailor your exercise program on a daily basis, depending on how you feel. During the first few weeks, you may notice that your heart beats faster and you breathe faster when you exercise, and your muscles feel tense afterward. You may feel more tired at night, but you're likely to sleep better and deeper than before. These are normal reactions to exercise that mean your body is adapting and getting into shape.

- Stop exercising right away if you have chest tightness or severe shortness of breath, or if you feel dizzy, faint, or sick to your stomach. If these symptoms occur, contact your doctor immediately. If you develop muscle pain or a cramp, gently rub and stretch the muscle. When the pain is gone, continue exercising with slow, easy movements. You may need to change your position or the way you are doing the exercise.

After Exercise

- Cool down after exercising. To cool down, simply do your exercise activity at a slower, more relaxed pace for three to five minutes. For instance, if you've been walking briskly, slow down to a stroll. Also do gentle stretches to avoid stiff or sore muscles the next day. This helps your body cool down, lets your heart slow down, and helps your muscles relax.

- Don't overstretch your muscles. Just stretch gently until you feel tension and then hold briefly.

- Massage any stiff or sore areas or apply heat or cold treatments to the area. Try soaking in a hot tub after working out–heat relaxes your joints and muscles and helps relieve pain. Cold also reduces pain and swelling for some people.

Make Exercise a Habit

We can all find many reasons not to exercise. Here are some of the most common reasons, along with some ways to overcome them.

"I haven't exercised in so long. What if I can't do it?"

It's normal to feel hesitant about something you haven't done for a while. To overcome such feelings, try not to think of exercise as competition with others or to compare what you're able to do now with what you used to be able to do. Instead, focus on your current abilities and do what you can. Think positively. Each accomplishment, no matter how small, will help reinforce your confidence.

"I'm out of shape. It will take too long to see results."

Often, long-term problems can be addressed and managed by setting goals and writing out a contract. Refer to the Goal Setting and Contracting information in Chapter 3, and follow those guidelines to make your own exercise contract.

"It hurts."

It's normal to have some soreness at first. Always remember to warm up beforehand and cool down afterward to help relax your muscles and reduce the pain. Also, remember that strengthening exercises, in the long run, are likely to reduce the pain of fibromyalgia. Other tips:

- Don't do vigorous exercises. If you notice a bit more pain or actually are unable to do as much as you have been, talk to your doctor or physical therapist about it.
- If just one or two areas of your body are painful, you can adapt your exercises to put less stress on those areas. For example, if you are having more pain in your lower body (the weight-bearing area), switch to water exercises or use a stationary bicycle without resistance instead of walking.

"My fibromyalgia is acting up."

When your fibromyalgia is very active and your pain is severe, don't skip your exercises entirely. Too much rest can be harmful, leading to stiffer and weaker muscles. Get plenty of rest, but also do range-of-motion exercises. They will help maintain your mobility. As your condition settles down, continue your range-of-motion exercises, and gradually get back to your regular program.

"I don't have enough time."

Follow an exercise schedule. Several short exercise periods are just as good as one long period. Choose times that will not conflict with work and family responsibilities that are important to you. Think of your exercise time as special time for yourself. Use this time to think about other creative goals for yourself.

Once you begin to get into shape, you may find that exercising actually seems to make more time for you. That's because when you have less pain, you're able to accomplish more in less time.

"It's boring."

Do exercises you enjoy. Listen to your favorite music or a audio book while exercising. Exercise with friends or family members who understand fibromyalgia. If you walk or bicycle, go to the park or another pleasant area.

"The weather's bad."

If you usually exercise with a group and can't get to your class, do your exercises at home. If you swim or walk, have a backup plan for indoor exercises when the weather is bad. For example, walk around a shopping mall if it's too cold or hot to walk outside. Have some exercise equipment or exercise videotapes at home.

"I don't like to exercise alone."

Ask friends or family members to exercise with you, or join an exercise class. Another option is to use one of the Arthritis Foundation's exercise videotapes to get the feeling of a group experience.

"It's too much work."

Maybe you're being too ambitious about your exercise program. Maybe you're trying to do too much. Relax! Enjoy the good feelings while you exercise and afterward. Exercising for fun is the best way to keep it up.

"My fibromyalgia isn't bothering me anymore."

Exercise probably has a lot to do with this. Instead of stopping, try some new and different exercises or activities that will vary your program or continue the same program.

CHAPTER ELEVEN

Eating Well

Does Food Affect Fibromyalgia?

Can what you eat cause, cure, or affect fibromyalgia? Since symptoms of fibromyalgia can vary from day to day, it's natural to think that what you ate yesterday may have caused or reduced the pain you feel today.

Research has not yet proven that any specific foods affect fibromyalgia, positively or negatively. But we do know for a fact that eating a good, balanced diet helps everyone's body function at its best. Following a balanced diet can help you feel better and stay healthy, prevent chronic diseases such as some cancers and cardiovascular disease, and be a positive step toward managing your fibromyalgia.
To adopt a healthier diet, concentrate on:

- reducing salt, fat, cholesterol, sugar, and alcohol
- adding or emphasizing variety, fiber, fruits and vegetables, calcium, and water.

Eating well does not mean you have to starve yourself or totally eliminate the foods you love. Rather, it means making small, gradual changes in what you eat to focus on healthful meals you enjoy. You are more likely to stick with these type of changes for good.

BENEFITS OF EATING WELL

- Helps you look and feel better;

- Reduces fatigue and maximizes energy;

- Helps prevent or lessen medication side effects;

- Helps avoid constipation and rids the body of waste products;

- Keeps the kidneys functioning properly;

- Maintains the chemical balance in our bodies.

A Note on Diet "Cures"

You may read or hear about claims that special diets, supplements, or foods cure health problems. Some are frauds. Others are unproven remedies (see Chapter 5). Consider diets unsafe and ineffective unless scientific tests prove them otherwise. Ask these questions: Does the diet eliminate any essential food group from the Food Guide Pyramid (discussed later in this chapter)? Does it stress only a few foods or eliminate others? If the answer is yes to either question, avoid the diet.

What Is a Good Diet?

Experts recommend seven basic guidelines for a balanced, healthful diet. You can use these guidelines in planning meals every day. The following sections explain how each of these guidelines is helpful to people in general.

GUIDELINES FOR A HEALTHFUL DIET

- Eat a variety of foods.

- Maintain a healthy weight.

- Use fat and cholesterol in moderation.

- Eat plenty of vegetables, fruits, and grain products.

- Use sugar in moderation.

- Use salt in moderation.

- If you drink alcohol, do so in moderation.

- Drink eight glasses of water a day.

Eat a Variety of Foods

Variety, balance, and moderation are keys to a healthful diet. Variety usually means eating more grains, fruits, and vegetables than most Americans do. A good diet includes some choices from each of five different groups of foods: breads and cereals, fruits, vegetables, dairy products, and meats. Eating a variety of foods gives you the 40 or more nutrients your body needs to grow and function.

Pain, fatigue, and depression can lower your appetite. Pain may cause you to avoid foods that require more time or effort to prepare. Follow the tips in the following box to make food preparation easier.

MAKE MEAL PREPARATION EASIER

- Plan rest breaks during meal preparation time.

- Use good posture while cooking.

- Keep the things you use most often out on the counter.

- Use convenience foods occasionally to reduce the strain of cooking meals.

- Add fresh fruit and bread to a frozen dinner to make a complete, satisfying meal.

- Purchase pre-sliced and chopped vegetables from the produce or frozen food sections of grocery stores.

- Use kitchen gadgets and appliances such as electric can openers and microwave ovens to make cooking tasks easier.

Health professionals in your community can help you learn more efficient cooking methods. Your doctor can refer you to an occupational therapist for advice on easier ways to cook. Some local chapters of the Arthritis Foundation and the Cooperative Extension Services of some state universities may also sponsor cooking classes or demonstrations with helpful hints for making cooking easier.

Some medications can also affect how well your body uses what you eat. For most people, eating a variety of foods will help keep up the levels of these nutrients. Talk to your physician about how the medications you take affect your nutritional status and whether a vitamin supplement may be useful for you.

Use Fat and Cholesterol in Moderation

Reducing fats, cholesterol, and salt in your diet may help prevent cardiovascular disease. Fat, a source of concentrated calories, contributes to extra pounds. To lower saturated fat and cholesterol, choose low-fat cuts of meat and low-fat dairy products. Reduce your servings of red meat and pork and limit the use of added fats, oils, salad dressings, nuts, and nut butters. A daily serving of meat or fish the size of a deck of playing cards (approximately 3 ounces) is adequate for most adults. Egg yolks should be limited to three per week.

Eat Plenty of Vegetables, Fruits, and Grain Products

Fruits, vegetables, and whole-grain products help give you energy and keep your bowels regular. Most of these foods are also low in fat, and are important sources of vitamins and nutrients. Starchy foods are high in complex carbohydrates, which help meet your body's energy needs. Foods high in carbohydrates are useful in weight control since they produce a feeling of fullness.

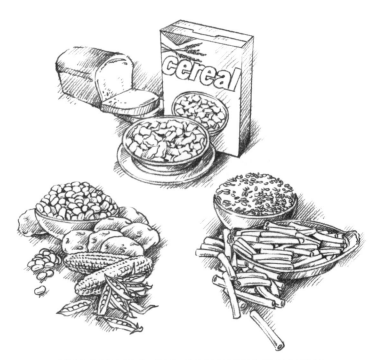

EXAMPLES OF STARCHY FOODS
Breads, Cereals
Rice, Beans
Pasta, Potatoes
Corn, Peas
Lima Beans

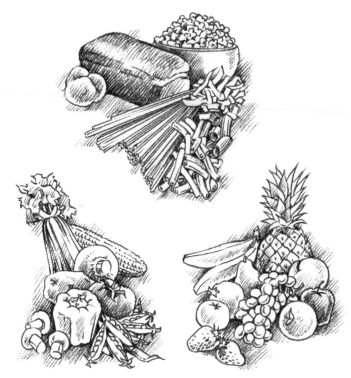

EXAMPLES OF HIGH-FIBER FOODS
Fruits
Vegetables
Whole-Grain Breads
Pasta, Popcorn

Fruits, vegetables, and whole-grain products are also excellent sources of fiber. Fiber comes from the parts of plants your body cannot digest. Some types of fibers result in softer stools and more rapid elimination of wastes. Foods with fiber can help you avoid constipation.

Some fibers such as oat bran help lower cholesterol levels. It is generally better to get fiber naturally from foods instead of from fiber supplements.

Use Sugar in Moderation

Sugar adds calories and promotes weight gain and tooth decay. When checking food labels for added sugar, look for the words *dextrose, sucrose, fructose, honey* and *dextrin.*

Use Salt (Sodium) in Moderation

Sodium causes your body to retain water, and can affect your blood pressure. Many foods now come with low- or no-salt-added choices. This makes it easier to maintain a low-sodium diet. However, watch levels on prepared food labels.

Drink Alcohol in Moderation

Excessive alcohol consumption can have many adverse effects on your health, including weakened bones, which can lead to osteoporosis. Alcohol also adds unwanted pounds with extra, empty calories. It can increase the uric acid in the body, increasing your susceptibility to gout.

Alcohol does not mix well with certain medications used in treating fibromyalgia. Alcohol can add to the sedative effect of tricyclic antidepressants and selective serotonin reuptake inhibitors (SSRIs), thereby causing temporary mental impairment. Stomach problems are more likely if you drink alcohol and take aspirin or other nonsteroidal anti-inflammatory drugs (NSAIDs). Large amounts of alcohol combined with acetaminophen can damage the liver. If you are taking any medications, check with your doctor or pharmacist about using alcohol, even in moderation.

The Food Guide Pyramid

The Food Guide Pyramid developed by the U.S. Department of Agriculture and Health and Human Services shows how to follow these dietary guidelines and make wise food choices. Select most foods from the bottom two layers of the pyramid and fewer foods from the top, based on the recommended number of servings. A variety of foods from the five major food groups should be eaten to help provide all the nutrients your body needs each day. The Food Guide Pyramid will help you eat a balanced diet with moderate amounts of sugar, sodium, and saturated fat. It will also help you get the right amount of calories to maintain a healthy weight.

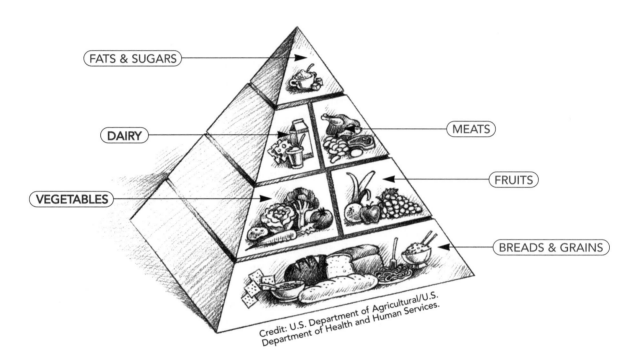

FATS & SUGARS

DAIRY

MEATS

VEGETABLES

FRUITS

BREADS & GRAINS

Credit: U.S. Department of Agricultural/U.S. Department of Health and Human Services.

Following the Food Guide Pyramid can help you eat a well-balanced diet that consists primarily of grains, fruits, and vegetables.

The Food Labeling Act

Beginning in 1994, a new nutrition label was required to appear on most foods. Many packages already listed ingredients, but there were no standards for comparing one food with another. The new label allows you to read the nutritional content of the food so you can make smart choices for a healthier diet.

Nutrition Facts

Serving Size 1 cup (30g)
Servings Per Container 12

Amount Per Serving

Calories 90	Calories from Fat 10

	% Daily Value*
Total Fat 1g	**2**%
Saturated Fat 0g	**0**%
Cholesterol 0mg	**0**%
Sodium 190mg	**8**%
Total Carbohydrate 22g	**7**%
Dietary Fiber 3g	**12**%
Sugars 9g	
Protein 3g	

Vitamin A	25%	Vitamin C	0%
Calcium	0%	Iron	25%

* Percent Daily Values are based on a 2,000 calorie diet. Your daily values may be higher or lower depending on your calorie needs:

	Calories	2,000	2,500
Total Fat	Less than	65g	80g
Sat Fat	Less than	20g	25g
Cholesterol	Less than	300mg	300mg
Sodium	Less than	2,400mg	2,400mg
Total Carbohydrate		300g	375g
Fiber		25g	30g

Calories per gram:
Fat 9 • Carbohydrate 4 • Protein 4

American Heart Association

The new food label makes it easier to compare food choices so you know what you're eating.

The Food Labeling Act also set new guidelines for health claims a food manufacturer can make. Claims such as "fat free," "cholesterol free," "low sodium," and others are now defined by government standards. Certain requirements must be met before these types of claims can be made. Instead of learning what each claim means, remember these key words to help you judge nutritional content:

- "Free" has the least amount.
- "Very low" and "Low" have a little more.
- "Reduced" or "Less" always means that the food has 25 percent less of that nutrient than the reference (or standard) version of the food.

Nutrition Resources

There are many sources for answers to your questions about diet. One place to start is with your doctor, who can refer you to experts in diet and nutrition for help with applying diet guidelines, planning a weight-loss program, or answering any of your questions.

Here are some other tips:

- Check with local hospitals, health clinics, and public health departments, which often have individual nutritional counseling and weight-reduction groups.
- See the Yellow Pages of the telephone directory under Nutritionists. Look for people who are registered dietitians or have a master's degree.
- Write to the Consumer Information Center, Pueblo, CO 80119, for a copy of "USDA's Food Guide Pyramid," a colorful, easy-to-read, 30-page booklet. (Cost is $1.)
- Contact the Cooperative Extension Service for answers to your questions about meal planning. Look under the "Government Offices" section of your phone book.
- Contact other voluntary health and professional organizations that promote a healthy diet, such as local chapters of the American Heart Association, American Cancer Society, American Diabetes Association, and American Dietetic Association.
- Check your bookstore or library for relevant, recently published books.

ON A PERSONAL NOTE

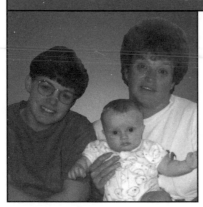

Gail Dunlop with her daughter and granddaughter

Thanks, Fibromyalgia
by Gail M. Dunlop
Valdese, NC

A fibromyalgia diagnosis doesn't mean the end of life—for me, it actually has signified a new beginning.

When the condition caused me to be unemployed for several years, I became bored and decided to return to school. Now, at age 45, I'm seeking an associate's degree in the arts with hopes of continuing my education by transferring to a university. Without this condition, I would not have attended college, particularly this late in life, and might never have discovered the thrill of putting words on paper, the joy of having something published, or my thirst for knowledge about literature and writing.

In addition to fueling my curiosity, attending school has boosted my self-esteem. While the routine classes and homework make me tired, they also give me a fulfilling sense of purpose and accomplishment. I've become friends with other older students as well as with younger ones who treat me as an equal. And school has also helped me stave off depression, a common problem for people with fibromyalgia.

I still have lots of pain (for which I take analgesics), and I walk with a cane—or two—because my legs ache constantly and tire quickly. But pursuing a goal and having the desire to succeed keep my spirits up. School has done more for my health than any pill I've swallowed.

*Reprinted from **Arthritis Today**, July/August 1996.*

CHAPTER TWELVE

Getting a Life— In Spite of Fibromyalgia

Key Aspects of a Wellness Lifestyle

If you have read Chapters 1 through 11 of this book, by now you realize that the key to living well with fibromyalgia is leading a healthy life—despite your disease. As you have read, that includes finding a healthy balance between exercise and rest, and eating a balanced, nutritious diet. It's also important to nourish your mind and spirit, as well as your body.

Consider the following keys to a healthy mental outlook.

Optimism

Having the view that things in general are pretty good can help you live longer and reduce your level of chronic stress. Expect good things to happen—and work toward them. Stop worrying so much! Live one day at a time and use relaxation techniques and healthy self-talk to counter pessimistic thoughts.

Humor

Laughter really is good medicine. Author Norman Cousins refers to laughing as "internal jogging." Anything that makes you smile brings relief to your mind and spirit. Some research has shown that humor may even improve your immune function.

Sense of Purpose

Do you believe that you have worth and that there is a purpose for your life and experiences? People who believe in themselves and in the meaning of their lives are happier, more satisfied, and serene. This belief in one's self is a choice that occurs regardless of life circumstances.

Sense of Control

Do you feel helpless or continually frustrated by your fibromyalgia or other challenges in your life? Given the same situation, some people will choose to feel helpless; others will feel a sense of control, a confidence that they can help influence their own well-being. Goal setting and contracting, problem solving, self-monitoring, keeping a journal, using communication skills to tell others about your needs, and planning are all ways to help you regain a sense of control.

Social Support

Is your life filled with satisfying relationships and love? Do you feel that others understand your fibromyalgia and the demands that it places on you? Are you getting the support that you need? Getting that support can be hard work. You need to be a friend to have a friend, and you need to be willing to listen to others as well as communicate your own needs in a clear, direct way.

Positive Self-Image

The way you feel about yourself is an important part of being healthy. Chronic pain and fatigue can drag you down and make you feel as if there's no point in taking care of yourself. Counteract negative feelings by being nice to yourself. You deserve it! Consider some of the following ways you might pamper yourself:

- Get your hair cut in a new style.
- Spring for a pedicure or manicure.
- Get a massage—this might not only lift your spirits but could also help alleviate pain.
- Start a book club or potluck supper group. It's an easy way to socialize with friends without all the labor involved in most kinds of entertaining.
- Rejuvenate in a long bubble bath.
- Adopt a pet from the local humane society. In addition to saving an animal's life, you'll bring some joy and companionship into your own.
- Pray or meditate.
- Help someone in some way.

WORK SHEET: THE BEST OF ME

List at least 10 qualities or aspects that make you unique, that you like or admire about yourself, and/or that you feel make you attractive (include at least one or two physical attributes).

1	
2	
3	
4	
5	
6	
7	
8	
9	
10	

Your Relationships with Others

Some experts believe that people with chronic conditions who don't have a strong support network are likely to have more pain, be less active, use more medication, and feel more depressed, helpless, and anxious than are people with a support network. Obviously, then, close relationships with others can have a positive effect on your psychological and physical well-being.

How well a family copes when faced with health problems depends greatly on their pre-fibromyalgia relationships. Some families pull closer together, united in their determination, and maintain an environment that is supportive of every member. Sadly, some families sag under the weight of a chronic illness and splinter apart.

How do the successful families manage?

- *Communication:* By sharing thoughts and feelings, family members better understand each other's expectations and needs.
- *Tolerance:* By maintaining respect for each other's limitations, family members are less likely to have emotional blowouts with each other.
- *Humor:* Like almost every other endeavor in life, a sense of humor can make any burden a little lighter.
- *Support:* Successful families are available to provide help and counsel regardless of circumstances.

Strong communication skills can be a vital tool in your relationships with your family and close friends, particularly now that fibromyalgia is part of the picture. The tips listed here will help you in all your dealings with loved ones, friends, business associates, or health-care professionals.

Communication: Using "I" Messages

Often when people are annoyed or frustrated with someone else, they express their feelings either too aggressively, thereby putting the recipient of the message on the defensive, or too passively, by clamming up and holding a grudge. It's easy to slip into using what psychologists call "you" messages: "Why do you always make us late?" "You don't understand how I feel." "You really make me angry when you do that."

"You" messages can be thought of as "verbal fists." The other person immediately feels under attack, and the natural reaction is to become defensive. Now both people have their verbal fists up, and the situation may escalate into an argument and bad feelings. Your message is lost in the transaction.

A better way to be heard is to use "I" messages. These are factual statements of how you feel; they don't accuse or blame the other person. When you say, "I get upset when I'm late," or "I am angry that you did that," the other person can respond to the content of what you've said, rather than defending against an attack.

Consider the following examples of "you" messages:

Friend 1: You're not helping! You're going to make us late. Can't you stay out of my way?

Friend 2: You're always complaining. You find fault with everything I do. You don't think of anyone but yourself.

Friend 1: Well, if you had the problems that I have, you wouldn't be so quick to criticize.

Now, consider the same messages that contain examples of "I" statements:

Friend 1: I really hate being late all the time. This disease gets in the way of everything I want to do. There must be some way to speed things up.

Friend 2: Your illness has changed things. I can see where it would be frustrating. It's difficult for me too, because I never know when offering help is the right thing to do.

Friend 1: I never realized that you felt this way. I can see how it could be confusing. I'll tell you what: If I need help in the future, I'll ask. Too much help makes me feel helpless.

Friend 2: That's a good solution. It will make me feel better too.

Listen to Yourself and Others

"I" messages take practice. Start by really listening and practice changing each "you" message you hear to an "I" message in your head. This mental exercise will soon translate to your own expressions.

Keep Trying

If "you" messages and assigning blame have been your typical way of communicating, the other person may not hear the "I" messages. Keep using them anyway, and eventually the other person will hear you.

Don't Manipulate

"I" messages should report honest feelings. When used to manipulate the other person, communication will get worse.

Express Positive Feelings, Too

"I" messages are wonderful for expressing positive feelings and compliments.

Learning to Listen

Listening is a crucial element of good communication, too. Many people are not good listeners because they don't know how to practice active listening. Active listening involves paying close attention to what another person is saying by making eye contact, leaning forward, and encouraging the speaker to continue with brief remarks like, "Mm-hm," or "Then what?"

Instead of responding with advice or information, first show that you understood the content of the other person's message by rephrasing, in your own words, what you think the speaker meant. If you've misunderstood what was said, this provides an immediate opportunity for correction. Acknowledge the person's emotional state, too. Simply saying, "You sound scared," or "I can see that you're angry," communicates your understanding, concern, and acceptance of the person's feelings. Often, this will encourage the speaker to talk even more openly.

Listening may be the single most important element in good communication. Many people are not good listeners because they assume listening is passive—they may hear the words but fail to understand the meaning. To become a good listener, you need to learn the skill of active listening. Here's what's involved in active listening:

- *Look interested.* Use nonverbal clues to show you're listening. Make eye contact, keep your posture relaxed, lean forward, use appropriate facial expressions (smile or look sympathetic), nod your head to show you are listening, touch the person (if appropriate).
- *Sound like you are interested.* Encourage the speaker to continue with brief phrases or words: "Mm-hm," "Oh?" "Go on," "Then what?" "Would you like to talk about it?"
- *Acknowledge the content.* In your own words, rephrase what you think the speaker meant. If this is not what the speaker was trying to communicate, you've provided the opportunity for correction.
- *Acknowledge the speaker's emotional state.* People communicate their feelings by tone of voice, facial expression, and other non-verbal cues. Simply saying "you sound sad/glad/angry/scared" communicates your understanding, concern, and acceptance of the person's feelings. Often this will encourage the speaker to talk even more openly.

Get the Data You Need!

A computer cannot process data it doesn't have—and neither can you! If you don't have enough information, you can't respond appropriately. How do you get the person to communicate further?

- *Ask for more data.* Be honest if you are confused or think you missed the point: "I don't understand." "Would you say that another way?" "How do you mean?" "Please expand on that." "Tell me more."
- *Ask about meaning.* Sometimes there's a gap between what a person says and what was meant. Paraphrasing is a good way to be sure you understood what the person meant. Be careful to paraphrase as a question, though. People don't like to be told what they meant. "You're telling me . . ." sounds like an accusation, and the response is likely to be anger or frustration because you didn't understand. "Are you saying . . .?" promotes further clarification.
- *Be specific.* We often speak in generalities when we actually need specifics. A question like "How do you feel?" may not elicit a very useful answer if what you really want to know is, "Are you upset?" or "Does your head still hurt?" or "Is the room warm enough?"

Sexuality and Fibromyalgia

Fibromyalgia can affect one's sexuality—which is not limited to just physical activity but also one's feelings of attractiveness, desire for emotional closeness, and openness to sensory experiences—in a number of ways. In fact, it's not unusual for a couple to experience communication and/or relationship difficulties when one partner has fibromyalgia. Part of the problem may stem from feelings of decreased self-esteem due to changes in physical capabilities. Feelings of depression may result in withdrawal from sexual activity. This withdrawal, if accompanied by a reluctance to discuss sexual needs and/or problems, can seriously jeopardize your relationship. Your partner may misinterpret withdrawal as rejection.

For men, especially, increased reliance on others for help can change a role as a main provider or caretaker to one that is more dependent upon other family members. Sexual problems may result.

To improve your sexual relationship with your partner, talk with your partner about your needs, desires, and ideas. Learn to use communication skills (see "Communication: Using 'I' Messages" in this chapter) to ask for what you need, to set boundaries, and to let your partner know what feels good to you. It is important that your partner express his or her feelings as well. Your partner may be concerned that sexual activity is painful for you and therefore is anxious about being intimate with you. Avoiding sex could create tension between you. Talking with one another honestly and regularly can help prevent this.

How Fibromyalgia Affects Sexuality

Fibromyalgia can cause a variety of physical problems that may affect sexuality. Here are some of the more common ones and some tips to minimize them:

Fatigue:
- Plan sexual activity for when you are rested.
- Plan ahead by pacing daily activities to avoid extreme fatigue.

Pain and Stiffness:
- Try stretching activities to reduce stiffness.
- Take a warm bath or shower before sexual relations to reduce pain.
- Find a more comfortable position.

Medications:
- Some medications can have side effects that affect sexuality. For example, some tranquilizers can suppress orgasms and desire for sex.
- Consult your doctor if you are concerned about medication side effects.

It is important to remember that there is no one right way to be sexually fulfilled. Having fibromyalgia may mean having to adapt your sexual activity, but it doesn't mean having to give up a close, intimate relationship with your partner.

TALKING WITH YOUR PARTNER ABOUT SEX

Fibromyalgia may affect how you feel about yourself sexually. Talking with your partner can help make you feel better and improve your partnership. Think about these questions and talk them over with your partner.

1. Has fibromyalgia altered your sexual relationship or your feelings about your sexuality?

2. What, if anything, has changed?

3. What is more or less the same?

4. Are there any sexual activities that are not as pleasant as they used to be?

5. Are there any that are more enjoyable?

6. Does lovemaking cause any certain problems for you or your partner?

7. Where on your body do you enjoy being touched and what areas do you find unpleasant?

8. Are there new things you would like to try? If so, what are they?

9. Have you talked to your partner about any of these things previously?

Adapted from Sexuality and MS, *National MS Society, 1983.*

Uplifting Activities

Consciously seeking out uplifting activities can help you balance out the hassles and problems that lead to stress, depression, pain, and fatigue. This means choosing to enjoy life by taking time out to have fun and enjoy yourself.

We aren't always taught how to nourish ourselves emotionally or spiritually. Sometimes, people are taught to do the exact opposite—to not express their emotions and feelings. Nourishment of the mind and spirit can take many forms, such as laughing, crying, singing, listening to music, meditating, praying, enjoying the beauty of nature, exercising, or reading inspirational and informational books. Use the Uplifts Scale in Chapter 8 to help you track events that make you feel good.

ACTIVITY: Things You Love to Do

Think about activities or things that you love to do, things that bring enjoyment and happiness to your life. These can be big things like taking a trip or little things like taking a bubble bath. Use the *Things I Love To Do* worksheet below to list these things. Try to come up with 15 items. Once you have a list, select your top five most enjoyable activities and build them into your schedule.

THINGS I LOVE TO DO

Write down as many activities as possible that bring you enjoyment and happiness. In the "Rank Top Five" column, indicate by number those five activities that you enjoy the most. In the "Last Time" column, indicate how long it has been since you engaged in each of your top five activities.

ACTIVITIES	RANK TOP FIVE (1-5)	LAST TIME
1.		
2.		
3.		
4.		
5.		
6.		
7.		
8.		
9.		
10.		
11.		
12.		
13.		
14.		
15.		

ACTIVITY: Targeting Your Time

Your use of time and your overall balance of activities can affect your health and satisfaction with life. Using the Time Target below, think about how satisfied you are with the time you now spend on key activities like hobbies, time alone or with friends, family time, and so on.

TARGETING YOUR TIME

Instructions: Read the names for each of the 12 activities listed in the wedges of the circle below. Think about how satisfied you are with the time you now spend on each activity. Color in the part of the wedge for each activity that best describes how that activity fits into your life. For example, if you are satisfied with time spent on an activity, color the center part of the wedge, in the "okay" section. Otherwise, indicate by coloring whether you "need less" or "need more" of the activity, or if the activity is "not important" in your life.

HOW CLOSE ARE YOU TO THE BULL'S-EYE?

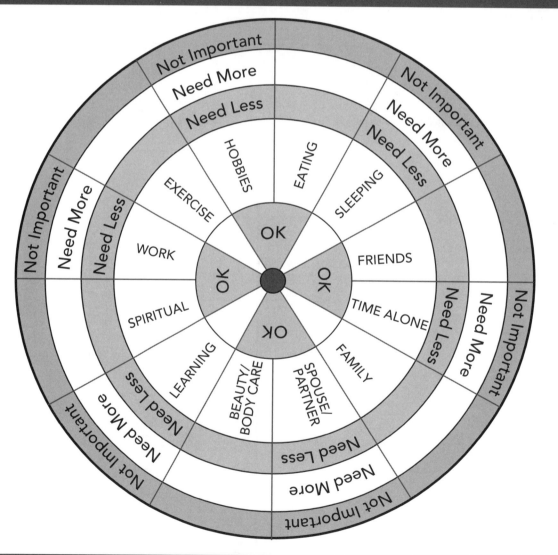

Follow the instructions on the Time Target work sheet. After you have completed the work sheet, look for any patterns. Is your life so balanced that most or all of the "bull's-eye" (the center circle) is colored in? Or do you have a lot of parts of the other circles colored in? Look for colored areas in these outer circles:

"Need Less" Circle

If you have a lot of this circle colored in, this may be a sign that you are having trouble setting priorities or saying "No." Are you feeling overwhelmed? If so, go back and read over the strategies for dealing with fatigue in Chapter 6.

"Need More" Circle

Is it hard for you to ask for what you need? Do you need more from people in relationships? Do you need to do better planning so you can spend more time on your more enjoyable activities? Remember to set goals, contract, problem solve, and plan to get where you want to be.

"Not Important"

If you have colored five or more of the activities as "not important," this may be a sign that you are feeling depressed. If you have lost interest in many activities that used to be pleasurable for you, if you've isolated yourself from friends, or if you feel like hurting yourself, seek professional help. Go back and review the signs of depression and suggestions for coping in Chapter 9.

There is no single solution to all the possible challenges that might be uncovered in a Time Target exercise. Be creative, use the skills you've learned throughout this book and other ideas you have to deal with them.

It is important to find those things in life that uplift and bring joy and happiness to your life. This can take time, patience, and determination, but if you can learn to balance out each of the hassles in your life with uplifting activities, fibromyalgia can become just a part of your life, not your whole life. Remember: Aim for the bull's-eye!

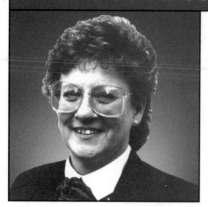

Talking to Yourself
by Ruth Kahn-Treadwell
Salem, OR

My body has fibromyalgia, but my mind doesn't. This presents a problem for the overachiever in me. My aches, pain, and fatigue tell me to stop what I'm doing, but at the same time I'm thinking about where I'd like to go and what I'd like to be doing.

The bridge between my body and soul seems to lie somewhere between denial and motivation. I call it "self-talk," and it helps me lead an almost normal life. I talk myself out of bed in the morning and into a warm shower. I dress myself comfortably and take my medication, knowing that some relief will come. I urge myself to go to my part-time job, thinking about the support and friendship I have there. (I might as well get paid while I'm not feeling well!) I also keep busy tutoring seniors about computers, teaching community education classes, and designing and painting decorative items to sell. I read voraciously and even make dinner most nights.

I refuse to give up a day in my life until I have given my body a fighting chance to perform. No, I don't feel much better than you do. I just refuse to give in to it.
*Reprinted from **Arthritis Today**, May/June 1996.*

A Final Word

What an accomplishment! Now that you've made this book your own by applying it to your own situation, you should be armed with the tools for living a better life with fibromyalgia. Before you go to work, let's review what these tools are and how they'll help you:

- **Getting the Facts.** If you have fibromyalgia, you've probably learned as much about the condition as possible. You know the most current research, have read the latest articles, have studied all the available reference material you could find on fibromyalgia, and constantly look for more information.

- **Managing Yourself.** Believing that you are the most important person in the management of your health is probably as important as learning about the condition itself. You now know what it takes to be a successful self-manager, and it is our hope that you have established personal goals for the self-management of your condition. If you sign a contract with yourself promising to fulfill these goals, you will be more likely to carry them out.

- **Managing Pain.** Because you have fibromyalgia, you know that pain can sometimes be a constant companion. But now you have a number of strategies to fight, block, or temporarily waylay your pain. Sometimes the pain will win the battles; sometimes you will. But, with your Pain-Management Plan in hand, in the end you will win the war.

- **Coping with Fatigue.** While fatigue may seem like the most taxing of all symptoms that accompany fibromyalgia, you now know that there are ways to manage your fatigue. Before you can do that, you know that it is important to understand what triggers your fatigue and what helps "perk you back up." Once you have a grasp on what's causing your fatigue, you'll have the knowledge needed to put your strategies for managing it into action.

- **Getting Better Sleep.** Probably the most frustrating aspect of living with fibromyalgia is how the condition interferes with your ability to sleep soundly. You now know what factors disturb sleep and ways to improve your sleep.

- **Exercising.** It may be hard to believe, but one of the best strategies to combat both the pain and fatigue you feel is to get off the couch and exercise. This is where you really get to apply your role as self-manager. Only you can see that you receive the proper amount of exercise that is needed to make you feel better and only you can know how much better that exercise makes you feel.

- **Getting Over Grief.** While fibromyalgia seems to take a toll on your body, at the same time your mind struggles against accepting the fact that this condition is part of your life. Once you reach a level of acceptance, you will be able to live well again, in spite of the changes fibromyalgia has made in your life.

- **Living Well.** Before you can truly live well with fibromyalgia, you will have to take steps toward healthy living in general. This includes keeping a positive attitude, having a sense of humor, managing your stress, eating a healthy diet, and getting plenty of exercise. It isn't always easy, and some days you'll want to ignore healthy-living tips. Just remember that when your body feels better, you'll feel better.

Glossary

acetaminophen: A type of pain reliever that does not contain aspirin and is available without a prescription under a variety of brand names.

acupressure: Application of pressure over specific muscle sites to relieve pain and muscle spasm.

acupuncture: A centuries-old method of pain relief used in China and introduced into America in recent years. Needles are used to puncture the body at sites associated with pain blockage.

acute pain: See *pain.*

adrenal glands: Glands located near the kidneys. These glands secrete *adrenaline*, a hormone that increases the heart rate and respiration rate when we feel frightened, threatened, or angry, preparing us to flee to safety or stand and fight. In people with fibromyalgia, this hormone is secreted abnormally. See also *hormones.*

adrenaline: See *adrenal glands.*

aerobic: An activity designed to increase oxygen consumption by the body, such as aerobic exercise or aerobic breathing.

alpha wave: A type of electrical wave produced by the brain during quiet wakefulness. Disturbance in the production of these and delta waves, which occur during deep sleep, is characteristic of disturbed sleep that is common in fibromyalgia.

American College of Rheumatology (ACR): An organization that provides a professional, educational, and research forum for rheumatologists across the country. Among its functions is helping determine what symptoms and signs define the various types of rheumatic disease diagnoses and what the appropriate treatments are for those diagnoses.

antidepressants: Medications used to relieve depression or sad moods. *Tricyclic antidepressants* may relieve nighttime muscle spasms in people with fibromyalgia. The term "tricyclic" refers to the basic chemical structure of this drug.

antihistamine: A drug that counteracts the action of histamine, a chemical produced in immune response (for example, when you have an allergic reaction to pollen). Histamine has powerful effects such as dilating blood vessels (thus lowering blood pressure) and stimulating secretion of gastric juices. These drugs also sometimes carry the side effect of drowsiness, a problem for people with fibromyalgia who are also battling fatigue.

anxiety: A state of being apprehensive, worried, or concerned.

apnea: See *sleep apnea.*

arthralgia: Pain in the joints in the absence of arthritis.

arthritis: From the Greek word "arth" meaning "joint," and the suffix "itis" meaning "inflammation." It generally means involvement of a joint from any cause, such as infection, trauma, or inflammation.

autoimmune disorder: An illness in which the body's immune system mistakenly attacks and damages tissues of the body. There are many types of autoimmune disorders, including arthritis and the rheumatic diseases.

biofeedback: a procedure that uses electrical equipment to help you be more aware of your body's reaction to stress and pain and to learn how to control your body's physical reactions. The equipment monitors your heart rate, blood pressure, skin temperature, and muscle tension. These body signals are shown on a screen or gauge so you can see how your body is reacting.

body leverage: Use of body weight, muscle strength, and joints to perform any physical task, such as lifting, pulling, or standing. Adapting ways of using body leverage increases efficiency and reduces muscle strain and pain.

body mechanics: The structures and methods with which your body moves and performs physical tasks.

bursa: A small sac located between a tendon and a bone. The bursae (plural for bursa) reduce friction and provide lubrication. See also *bursitis.*

bursitis: Inflammation of a bursa, which can occur when the joint has been overused or when the joint has become deformed by arthritis. Bursitis makes it painful to move or put pressure on the affected joint.

capsaicin: A chemical contained in some hot peppers. Capsaicin gives these peppers their "burn" and has painkilling properties. It is available in nonprescription creams that can be rubbed on the skin over a joint to relieve pain.

chronic fatigue syndrome (CFS): A condition manifested by long-term fatigue. The symptoms of CFS and fibromyalgia are similar, but people with CFS don't experience the pain that is characteristic of fibromyalgia.

chronic pain: See *pain.*

chronobiology: Study of the timing, rhythms, and cycles of biological events such as ovulation, secretion of hormones, or temperature fluctuations.

circadian rhythm: The daily, monthly, and seasonal schedules on which living things carry out essential biological tasks, such as eating, digesting, eliminating, growing, and resting. Disruption of these rhythms, as when you must travel rapidly across time zones (promoting jet lag), has a negative and sometimes profound impact on performance and mood.

continuous positive airway pressure: See *CPAP*.

control group: A group of people used as a standard for comparison in scientific studies. For example, a scientist who wants to know if daytime sleepiness is linked with fibromyalgia might study the amount of sleepiness experienced during a year in two groups: women with fibromyalgia (the study group) and women without fibromyalgia (the control group).

cool-down exercises: A series of physical activities that allow your heart and respiration rates to return to normal after being elevated by exercise.

corticosteroids: A hormone produced in your body and related to cortisone. Corticosteroids can also be synthetically produced (that is, made in a laboratory) and have powerful anti-inflammatory affects. These are not the same as the dangerous performance-enhancing drugs that some athletes use to promote strength and endurance.

cortisone: A hormone produced by the cortex of the adrenal gland. Cortisone has potent anti-inflammatory effects but can also have side effects.

costochondritis: Tenderness or pain in the tissue covering the rib cage and under the breasts. May be a feature of fibromyalgia.

CPAP: Stands for *continuous positive airway pressure,* a method of keeping the nasal airway open in people who experience chronic breathing obstruction during sleep.

deconditioning: Loss of muscle mass and strength because of inactivity. See also *reconditioning*.

deep breathing: Drawing air into the lungs, filling them as much as possible, and then exhaling slowly. Performing this type of breathing rhythmically for a few minutes increases the amount of oxygen refreshing your brain and produces relaxation and readiness for mental tasks.

delta sleep: Deep, restorative sleep; a period of sleep in which a unique type of brain wave, called the delta wave, is produced by the brain. Certain vital body functions occur during delta sleep. Disturbances of delta sleep are characteristic of fibromyalgia.

delta wave: A type of brain wave produced during deep sleep. See also *delta sleep*.

depression: A state of mind characterized by gloominess, dejection, or sadness.

disease: Sickness. Some physicians use this term only for conditions in which a structural or functional change in tissues or organs has been identified.

disorder: An ailment; an abnormal health condition.

distraction: To deliberately shift your attention from a distressing experience or sensation and to focus on a pleasant or neutral one, for the purpose of relieving anxiety, stress, or pain. For example, if you have fibromyalgia pain, you might focus on a favorite piece of art, music, or remembrance of a happy moment instead of the pain.

double-blind studies: A method used in scientific studies to compare one intervention (such as a new medication) with other interventions, sometimes including no intervention. In this method, the study participants and the persons evaluating the interventions are "blinded"–that is, they aren't told who is getting the intervention that is being tested–so their responses will not be influenced by their opinions or expectations of the intervention.

electrical stimulation: see *biofeedback* and *TENS*.

endorphins: Natural painkillers produced by the human nervous system and having qualities similar to opiate drugs. Endorphins are released during exercise and when we laugh.

endurance exercises: Exercises such as swimming, walking, and cycling that use the large muscles of the body and are dependent on increasing the amount of oxygen that reaches the muscles. These exercises strengthen muscles and increase and maintain physical fitness.

enkephalins: Molecular components of proteins. Enkephalins carry and manage messages in the brain and spinal cord and play a part in pain perception, movement, mood, behavior, and regulation of release of some hormones.

ergonomics: The study of human capabilities and limitations in relation to the work system, machine, or task, as well as the study of the physical, psychological, and social environment of the worker. Also known as "human engineering."

exercise physiologists: Health professionals who apply their knowledge of basic physical and chemical processes in the human body to evaluation of the effects and benefits of exercise. An exercise physiologist is qualified to develop individualized programs of appropriate exercise for people with fibromyalgia, arthritis, and other rheumatic diseases.

fatigue: A general worn-down feeling of having no energy. Fatigue can be caused by excessive physical, mental, or emotional exertion, by lack of sleep, and by inflammation or disease.

fibromyalgia: A noninfectious rheumatic condition affecting the body's soft tissue. Characterized by muscle pain, fatigue, and non-restorative sleep, fibromyalgia has no associated abnormal X-ray or laboratory findings. It is often associated with headaches and irritable bowel syndrome.

fibrositis: An out-of-date name for *fibromyalgia*. Since the "itis" part of this term denotes inflammation, which is absent in fibromyalgia, physicians are dropping the term "fibrositis."

flare: A flare is a term used to describe the times when the disease or condition is at its worst.

flexibility exercises: Muscle stretches and other activities designed to maintain flexibility and to prevent stiffness or shortening of ligaments and tendons.

Food Guide Pyramid: An illustration (see Chapter 11) developed by the U.S. Department of Agriculture to represent the types and proportions of foods that are needed each day for a healthy diet.

Food Labeling Act: Recent legal decree of the U.S. government, mandating the type of information that must be given on food labels regarding nutritional content. This Act ensures that consumers will have easy-to-read fat, protein, fiber, carbohydrate, and calorie content information, and more.

gate theory: A theory of how pain signals travel to the brain. According to this theory, pain signals must pass a "pain gate" that can be opened or closed by various positive (e.g., feelings of happiness) or negative (e.g., feelings of sadness) factors.

genetic predisposition: Susceptibility to a specific disease or illness caused by certain genetic (inherited) characteristics.

good posture: The most efficient and least stressful body position for standing, walking, sitting, working, and reclining.

grief: Feelings of loss; acute sorrow.

guided imagery: A method of managing pain and stress. Following the voice of a "guide," an audiotape or videotape, or one's own internal voice, attention is focused on a series of images that lead one's mind away from the stressor or pain.

hormones: Concentrated chemical substances produced in the glands or organs and having specific—and usually multiple—regulatory effects to carry out in the body. See also *adrenaline, hypothyroidism, neural hormones, pituitary (gland), serotonin, steroids.*

hyperparathyroidism: A condition due to an increase in the secretions of the parathyroid gland, causing bone changes and elevated levels of calcium and decreased levels of phosphorus in the blood. Hyperparathyroidism may be associated with musculoskeletal pain.

hypothalamic-pituitary-adrenal (HPA) axis: One of the main brain-hormonal stress response axes (i.e., places where brain function and hormonal function are coordinated in response to stress).

hypothalamus: A portion of the brain, buried deep within the skull, that has a regulatory role in many of your body's most vital functions, including progression through the stages of sleep.

hypothyroidism: Diminished production of thyroid hormone. This causes the body to slow down in the way it stores and uses energy, resulting in fatigue, a tendency to gain weight, excessive sleep need, and sometimes muscle pains. See also *hormones.*

ICF-1: See *somatomedin C.*

illness: Poor health; sickness.

immune response: Activation of the body's immune system.

immune system: Your body's very complex biochemical system for defending itself against bacteria, viruses, wounds, and other injuries. Among the many components of the system are a variety of cells (such as T cells), organs (such as the lymph glands), and chemicals (such as histamine and prostaglandins).

inflammation: A response to injury or infection that involves a sequence of biochemical reactions. Inflammation can be generalized, causing fatigue, fever, and pain, or tenderness all over the body. It can also be localized, for example, in joints, where it causes redness, warmth, swelling, and pain. Inflammation is not a symptom of fibromyalgia.

internist: A physician who specializes in internal medicine; sometimes called a primary-care physician.

irritable bowel syndrome: A chronic, noninflammatory disease that gives no clues, such as changes in cell structure, as to its cause. Symptoms include abdominal pain, painless diarrhea, constipation, and sometimes alternating bouts of diarrhea and constipation.

isometric exercises: Exercises that build the muscles around joints by tightening the muscles without moving the joints.

isotonic exercises: Exercises that strengthen muscles by moving the joints.

juvenile primary fibromyalgia syndrome: Fibromyalgia in children.

lactose intolerance: Inability to properly digest lactose, which is contained in milk.

lupus (systemic lupus erythematosus): The term used to describe an inflammatory connective tissue autoimmune disease that can involve the skin, joints, kidneys, blood, and other organs and is associated with antinuclear antibodies.

massage: A technique of applying pressure, friction, or vibration to the muscles, by hand or using a massage appliance, to stimulate circulation and produce relaxation and pain relief.

massage therapist: One who has completed a program of study and is licensed to perform massage.

meditation: A sustained period of deep inward thought, reflection, and openness to inspiration.

metabolism: Your body's continuous chemical and physical processes, consisting of building up (creating new body tissue from food) and breaking down (deriving energy and creating waste products from tissue).

migraine (headache): A severe, throbbing headache, often recurring, that begins with spasm or constriction of the arteries in the skull. Migraine headaches are often accompanied by nausea and vomiting and sensitivity to light and sound.

morbidity (rate): The frequency or proportion of people with a particular diagnosis or disability in a given population.

myalgia: Pain of the muscles.

myofascial pain syndrome: Describes a localized area of muscle and surrounding tissue pain or tenderness.

narcotic: A class of drugs that reduce pain by blocking pain signals traveling from the central nervous system to the brain. While narcotics have the potential to be addictive and are abused by some people, they can be used very safely for effective pain relief under skilled medical supervision.

neural hormones: Hormones produced in the brain and central nervous system. See also *hormones.*

nocturnal myoclonus: A benign type of seizure activity that occurs, usually as a sudden jerk or thrash of the leg, in the period of transition to sleep. These occur in many people in the general population as well as in people with fibromyalgia, and they may disrupt sleep.

nonrestorative sleep: See *stages of sleep.*

NSAID (nonsteroidal anti-inflammatory drug): A type of drug that does not contain steroids but is used to relieve pain by reducing inflammation.

objective: Capable of being observed or measured; for example, infection can be objectively observed by the presence of bacteria in a blood test or culture test. See also *subjective*.

obstructive sleep apnea: See *sleep apnea*.

osteoarthritis: A disease causing cartilage breakdown in certain joints (spine, hands, hips, knees) resulting in pain and deformity.

pacing: Scheduling your daily tasks so that heavy and light tasks are alternated and work is balanced with rest.

pain: A sensation or perception of hurting, ranging from discomfort to agony, that occurs in response to injury, disease, or functional disorder. Pain is your body's alarm system, signaling that something is wrong. *Acute* pain is temporary and related to nerve endings stimulated by tissue damage and improves with healing. *Chronic* pain may be mild to severe but persists due to prolonged tissue damage or due to pain impulses keeping the gate open.

pediatrician: A physician who has taken special training and specializes in the diagnosis, treatment, and prevention of childhood and adolescent illness.

pediatric rheumatologist: See *rheumatologist*.

peptic ulcer: A benign (not cancerous) lesion in the stomach or duodenum that may cause pain, nausea, vomiting, or bleeding. Such lesions can be caused by nonsteroidal anti-inflammatory drugs such as aspirin or ibuprofen.

perceived exertion: An individual's subjective measure of how much effort is required to perform a task.

physiatrist: A physician who takes additional training after medical school and specializes in the field of physical medicine and rehabilitation.

physical therapist: A person who has taken professional training and is licensed in the practice of physical therapy.

physical therapy: Methods and techniques of rehabilitation to restore function and prevent disability following injury or disease. Methods used may include applications of heat and cold, assistive devices, massage, and an individually tailored program of exercises.

pituitary (gland): A small gland, located at the base of the brain, which secretes pituitary hormones. These hormones play a vital role in growth and development, how the body stores and uses energy, and the activity of other glands. See also *hormones*.

podiatrist: A health professional who specializes in care of the foot. Formerly called a chiropodist.

prioritizing: Choosing the most important activities or responsibilities; placing tasks in order so that your attention goes first to those that are most important or pressing.

progressive relaxation: A method of relieving muscle tension by focusing on one body part, then another, in sequence, usually beginning with the muscles of the toes and feet and ending with the facial muscles.

psychiatrist: A physician who has taken additional training after medical school in the study, treatment, and prevention of mental disorders. A psychiatrist may provide counseling and prescribe medicines and other therapies.

psychologist: A trained professional, usually a PhD rather than an MD, who specializes in the mind and mental processes, especially in relation to human and animal behavior. A psychologist may measure mental abilities and provide counseling.

psychosomatic: Pertaining to the link between the mind (psyche) and the body (soma). This term once suggested something negative ("You're not sick, it's all in your head"); however, as we grow to understand the mind and body connection more fully, the word is taking on new meaning.

range of motion: The distance and angles at which your joints can be moved, extended, and rotated in various directions. Full or normal range of motion means that the joints move without impairment to their normal limits up, down, around, forward, and back. Limited range of motion means that stiffness, pain, or other problems interfere with free movement.

rapid eye movement (REM) sleep: The period of sleep in which people dream, occurring about every 90 minutes during normal sleep. It gets its name from rapid eye movements that occur under the closed lids during this period. Scientists think that storage of information in long-term memory may also occur during REM sleep. See also *stages of sleep* and *restorative sleep*.

Raynaud's phenomenon: Restriction of blood flow to the fingers, toes, or (rarely) to the nose or ears, in response to cold or emotional upset. This results in temporary blanching or paleness of the skin, tingling, numbness, and pain.

reconditioning: Restoring or improving muscle tone and strength with appropriate and balanced exercise, nutrition, and rest. See also *deconditioning.*

relaxation: A state of release from mental or physical stress or tension.

REM: See *rapid eye movement (REM) sleep.*

remission: The term used to describe the period of time when the symptoms of a disease or condition improve or even disappear altogether.

repetitive strain injury: Pain caused by repeated muscle use.

restless legs syndrome: Peculiar "crawling" or spastic sensations in the legs that produce a need to move the legs; often worse in evenings.

restorative sleep: See *stages of sleep.*

rheumatic disease: A general term referring to conditions characterized by pain and stiffness of the joints or muscles. The American College of Rheumatology currently recognizes over 100 rheumatic diseases. The term is often used interchangeably with "arthritis" (meaning joint inflammation), but not all rheumatic diseases affect the joints or involve inflammation.

rheumatoid arthritis: A chronic, inflammatory autoimmune disease in which the body's protective immune system turns on the body and attacks the joints, causing pain, swelling, and deformity.

rheumatologist: A physician who has taken additional training after medical school and specializes in the diagnosis, treatment, and prevention of arthritis and other rheumatic disorders. *Pediatric rheumatologist:* A rheumatologist who specializes in the diagnosis, treatment, and prevention of arthritis or other rheumatic diseases in children and adolescents.

self-help: Any course, activity, or action that you do for yourself to improve your circumstances or ability to cope with a situation.

self-talk: That "little voice in your head" you use to talk to yourself, out loud or in thought. When self-talk is positive, the voice is like a cheering section. When it's stuck in negative patterns, the voice criticizes your every action or predicts failure for every enterprise.

serotonin: A hormone that constricts blood vessels and contracts smooth muscle. See also *hormones, migraine (headache), SSRI, stages of sleep.*

skeletal muscles: The voluntary muscles that are involved primarily in moving parts of the body. "Voluntary" in this sense refers to the muscles that move in response to our decisions to walk, bend, grasp, and so on, as opposed to muscles such as the heart, which do their work without our willful direction.

sleep apnea: Cessation of breathing during sleep, caused by obstruction of the nasal airway, sometimes many times during the night. This condition is associated with obesity, but not all people who have sleep apnea are obese. Because the brain must arouse the sleeper from deep sleep to relieve the obstruction and restore breathing, sleep apnea has serious health effects.

social worker: A person who has taken professional training and is licensed to assist people in need by helping them capitalize on their own resources and connecting them with social services (for example, home nursing care or vocational rehabilitation).

soft-tissue rheumatism: Pertaining to the many rheumatic conditions affecting the soft (as opposed to the hard or bony) tissues of the body. Fibromyalgia is one type of soft-tissue rheumatism. Others are bursitis, tendinitis, and focal myofascial pain.

somatomedin C (also called ICF-1): A hormone produced by the liver in response to growth hormone stimulation. Somatomedin C stimulates repair of muscle, bone, and skin.

SSRI (selective serotonin reuptake inhibitor): A recently developed group of medications used to treat depression, including Prozac and Zoloft. These work by decreasing levels of serotonin in the brain and are sometimes better tolerated and perhaps more effective than other antidepressants.

stages of sleep: Four phases that occur and reoccur during a normal night of sleep, each characterized by specific types of brain wave activity. Stage 1 is a transition state between wakefulness and sleep. Stage 2 is the first level of true sleep. Stages 3 and 4 are the deepest, most restorative stages. *Restorative sleep* is sleep in which Stages 3 and 4 occur uninterrupted and that promotes renewal of health or sleep. *Nonrestorative sleep* is sleep in which Stage 3 or 4 sleep is interrupted, shortened, or denied, thus denying the restorative benefits as well. See also *alpha wave, delta wave,* and *rapid eye movement (REM) sleep.*

steroids: A group name for lipids (fat substances) produced in the body and sharing a particular type of chemical structure. Among these are bile acids, cholesterol, and some hormones. Not the same as anabolic steroids, drugs synthesized from testosterone (the male sex hormone), and used by some athletes to promote strength and endurance.

strain: Injury to a muscle, tendon, or ligament by repetitive use, trauma, or excessive stretching.

strengthening exercises: Exercises that help maintain or increase muscle strength. See also *isometric exercises* and *isotonic exercises.*

stress: The result produced when the body is acted upon by excessive physical or emotional forces. The term is commonly used to denote either a cause or an effect.

subjective: Events or circumstances that are measured through one's personal perceptions but cannot be verified by objective measures. For example, pain in fibromyalgia can be felt and described but cannot be measured with a blood test, an X-ray, or other tests. See also *objective.*

substance P: A molecule produced in the spinal cord in response to injury. Substance P stimulates nerve endings and produces pain, thus notifying the brain of injury and imminent danger.

sustained pain: See *pain.*

syndrome: A collection of symptoms and/or physical findings that characterize a particular abnormal condition or illness.

target heart rate: The number of heartbeats per minute that people want to reach during exercise in order to gain maximum benefits. Because the normal heart rate changes as we age, target heart rates are grouped by age.

tender-point injection: Injection of a painkilling medication directly into a tender point that is causing acute or persistent pain. Though the injection is painful, it can lead to local pain relief lasting from hours to several months.

tender points: Areas in the body that are abnormally sensitive, causing pain when pressed. People with fibromyalgia have tender points in certain areas of the body. Presence of these tender points helps in the diagnosis of fibromyalgia. Also called *trigger points.*

tendinitis: Inflammation of a tendon.

tendon: A cord of dense, fibrous tissue uniting a muscle to a bone.

tennis elbow: Irritation or strain of the muscles that attach to the lateral side of the elbow. This may be caused by repetitive action, like that of swinging a tennis racket.

TENS: a treatment for pain that involves a small device that directs mild electric pulses to nerves in the painful area.

tension headaches: Headaches caused by states of mental, nervous, or muscular strain or stress.

tissue: A collection of similar cells that act together to perform a specific function in the body. The primary tissues are epithelial (skin), connective (ligaments and tendons), bone, muscle, and nervous.

TMJ (temporomandibular joint) syndrome: A painful syndrome involving the hinge joints of the jaw, in front of the earlobes. It may be due to arthritis of the joint or due to pain of surrounding muscles. May also be called "TMJ dysfunction."

tranquilizer: A type of drug with a calming, soothing effect that can help reduce anxiety and painful muscle tension and spasms.

tricyclic antidepressants: See *antidepressants*.

trigger point: See *tender points*.

trigger-point injection: See *tender-point injection*.

trochanteric bursitis: Irritation of the trochanteric bursa, which is located on the bony prominence of the femur or thigh. See also *bursitis*.

ultrasound: A method for treating pain that uses high-energy sound waves to bring comfort to painful joints and muscles. A physical or occupational therapist must perform this technique.

unproven remedies: Any treatments that are not yet proven safe and effective through repeated scientific studies involving adequate numbers of people. May include health frauds that have no scientific basis for their claims or experimental treatments still under study.

visualization: A method of thinking that engages the imagination to help you achieve a goal. To meet a practical goal, such as making an important sale, you might visualize a meeting in which the sales pitch will be made. To achieve an abstract goal, such as feeling more cheerful on a gloomy day, you might picture yourself getting out of bed and putting on a favorite outfit.

vivid imagery: Mental pictures with strong emotional associations.

warm-up: Gentle movement to warm up the muscles before performing stretches and more strenuous exercise.

Bibliography

The following resources were used in preparation of this book.

Arthritis Foundation. *Fibromyalgia Self-Help Course, class participant's manual.* Atlanta, GA, 1995.

Arthritis Foundation. *Fibromyalgia Self-Help Course, course leader's manual.* Atlanta, GA, 1995.

Arthritis Foundation. *Primer on the Rheumatic Diseases. 10th ed.* Atlanta, GA, 1993.

Bennett, Robert M. "The Fibromyalgia Syndrome: Myofascial Pain and the Chronic Fatigue Syndrome." In *Textbook of Rheumatology, 4th ed., vol. 1,* eds. W. N. Kelley, E. D. Harris Jr., S. Ruddy, and C. B. Sledge. Philadelphia, PA: W. B. Saunders Co., 1993, pp. 471-483.

Bennett, Robert M., Sharon R. Clark, Stephen M. Campbell, and Carol S. Burckhardt. "Low Levels of Somatomedin C in Patients with the Fibromyalgia Syndrome." *Arthritis & Rheumatism,* Vol. 35, No. 10, Oct. 1992, p. 1113.

Bloomfield S. A., and E. F. Coyle. "Bed rest, detraining, and retention of training-induced adaptation." In *ACSM's resource manual for guidelines for exercise testing and prescription,* eds. J. L. Durstine, A. C. King, P. L. Painter, J. L. Roitman, and L. D. Zwiren. Philadelphia, PA: Lea and Febiger, 1993, pp. 115-128.

Boisset-Pioro, H. Mathilde, MD, CM; John M. Esdaile, MD, MPH; and Mary-Ann Fitzcharles, MD. "Sexual and Physical Abuse in Women with Fibromyalgia Syndrome." *Arthritis & Rheumatism,* Vol. 38, No. 2, Feb. 1995, pp. 235-241.

Burns, David, MD. *Feeling Good: The New Mood Therapy.* A Signet Book, 1980.

Carette, Simon. "Chronic Pain Syndromes." *Annals of the Rheumatic Diseases,* Vol. 55, 1996, pp. 497-501.

Conn, Doyt L., MD. "Searching for a Top Doc? Don't Go by the Book." *Arthritis Today,* Nov.-Dec. 1996, p. 32.

Dorland's Illustrated Medical Dictionary. 28th ed. Philadelphia, PA: W. B. Saunders Co., 1994.

Dunkin, Mary Anne. "Fibromyalgia Comes Out of the Closet." *Arthritis Today,* Sept.-Oct. 1993, pp. 24-28.

Dunkin, Mary Anne, ed. "New Clues to the Cause of Fibromyalgia." *Arthritis Today.* Mar.-Apr. 1993, p. 10.

Educational Rights for Children with Arthritis-Related Conditions publication. Atlanta, GA: Arthritis Foundation, 1996.

Fransen, RN, Jenny, and I. Jon Russell, MD. *The Fibromyalgia Help Book: Practical Guide to Living Better with Fibromyalgia.* St. Paul, MN: Smith House Press, 1996.

Hench, MD, P. Kahler. "Sleep and Rheumatic Disease." *Bulletin on the Rheumatic Diseases,* Vol. 45, No. 8, Dec. 1996. pp. 1-5.

Hudson, James I., MD, and Harrison G. Pope Jr., MD. "Does Childhood Sexual Abuse Cause Fibromyalgia?" *Arthritis & Rheumatism,* Vol. 38, No. 2, Feb. 1995, pp. 161-163.

Kelley, W. N., Ed Harris Jr., S. Ruddy, and C. B. Sledge, eds. *Textbook of Rheumatology. 5th ed.* Philadelphia, PA: W. B. Saunders Co., 1997.

Kubler-Ross, E. *On Death and Dying.* New York: Macmillan Publishing Co., 1981.

National Arthritis Data Workgroup, unpublished data, 1997.

Pennebaker, MD, James W. *Opening Up: The Healing Power of Confiding in Others.* New York: Avon Books, 1990.

Physician's Desk Reference. 50th ed. Montvale, NJ: Medical Economics Co., 1996.

Potera, Carol. "Fibromyalgia Finding." *Arthritis Today*, Jan.-Feb. 1995, p. 9.

Russell, I. J., J. E. Michalek, G. A. Vipraio, E. M. Fletcher, M. A. Javors, and C. A. Bowden. "Platelet 3H-Imipramine Uptake Receptor Density and Serum Serotonin Levels in Patients with Fibromyalgia/ Fibrositis Syndrome." *Journal of Rheumatology.* Vol. 19, 1992, pp. 104-109.

Russell I. J., H. Vaeroy, M. Javors, and F. Nyberg. "Cerebrospinal Fluid Biogenic Amine Metabolites in Fibromyalgia/Fibrositis Syndrome and Rheumatoid Arthritis." *Arthritis and Rheumatism,* Vol. 35, 1992, pp. 550-556.

Russell I. J., G. A. Vipraio, E. M. Fletcher, Y. M. Lopez, M. D. Orr, and J. E. Michalek. "Characteristics of Spinal Fluid, Substance P and Calcitonin Gene Related Peptide in Fibromyalgia Syndrome." *Arthritis and Rheumatism.* 39(9supp): Abstract 1485.

Simms, MD, Robert W. "Fibromyalgia Syndrome: Current Concepts in Pathophysiology, Clinical Features, and Management." *Arthritis Care and Research,* Vol. 9, No.4, Aug. 1996, pp. 315-328.

Stedman's Medical Dictionary, 25th Ed., Illustrated. Baltimore, MD: Williams & Wilkins, 1990.

Taylor, Mary Lou, PhD, Dana R. Trotter, MD, and M. E. Csuka, MD. "The Prevalence of Sexual Abuse in Women with Fibromyalgia." *Arthritis & Rheumatism*, Vol. 38, No. 2, Feb. 1995, pp. 229-234.

Textbook of Rheumatology. 3rd ed. Philadelphia, PA: W. B. Saunders Co., 1990.

Webster's New World Dictionary. 3rd College ed. New York: Simon & Schuster, Inc., 1988.

Wolfe, Frederick, Kathryn Ross, Janice Anderson, I. Jon Russell, and Liesi Hebert. "The Prevalence and Characteristics of Fibromyalgia in the General Population." *Arthritis and Rheumatism,* Vol. 38, No. 1, Jan. 1995, pp. 19-28.

Yunus, M. B., and A. T. Masic. "Juvenile Primary Fibromyalgia Syndrome: A Clinical Study of Thirty-Three Patients and Matched Normal Controls." *Arthritis and Rheumatism*, Vol. 28, 1985, pp. 138-145.

Resources

Suggested Fibromyalgia Materials List

This list of fibromyalgia materials and resources was developed by the Arthritis Foundation to assist people with fibromyalgia. A review committee, made up of Arthritis Foundation chapter program directors and heads of fibromyalgia organizations, was involved in the selection process. Resources on the enclosed list were included or excluded solely at their combined suggestion. Resources include both Arthritis Foundation and non-Arthritis Foundation materials. These are not however, Arthritis Foundation-reviewed materials.

Although all the materials on this list are being used by various Arthritis Foundation chapters, their inclusion here does *not* imply Arthritis Foundation endorsement. Neither does the exclusion of a resource imply that it is not usable, merely that it was not a material with which many of the reviewers were familiar.

We hope this list will provide a starting point in your education on fibromyalgia.

Books

Backstrom, Gayle, with Bernard R. Rubin, DO. *When Muscle Pain Won't Go Away: The Relief Handbook for Fibromyalgia and Chronic Muscle Pain.* Dallas, TX: Taylor Publishing Co., 1995.

Cousins, Norman. *Anatomy of an Illness: As Perceived by the Patient.* New York, NY: W.W. Norton & Co., 1979.

Cousins, Norman. *The Healing Heart.* New York, NY: W. W. Norton & Co., 1983.

Fransen, RN, Jenny, and I. Jon Russell, MD. *The Fibromyalgia Help Book: Practical Guide to Living Better with Fibromyalgia.* St. Paul, MN: Smith House Press, 1996.

Fries, MD James F. *Arthritis: A Take Care of Yourself Health Guide.* Reading, MA: Addison-Wesley Publishing, 1995.

Goldstein, MD, Jay A. *Betrayal by the Brain: The Neurological Basis of Chronic Fatigue Syndrome, Fibromyalgia Syndrome and Related Neural Disorders.* Binghamton, NY: Haworth Press, Inc., 1996.

Greenburg, MD, M., and L. Frank, MD. *Doctor, Why Do I Hurt So Much?* Minneapolis, MN: DCI/Chronimed Publishing, 1992.

Kabat-Zinn, PhD, Jon. *Full Catastrophe Living.* New York, NY: Dell Publishing, 1990.

Klippel, MD, John H., Cornelia Weyand, MD and Robert Wortmann, MD, eds. *Primer on the Rheumatic Diseases*, 11th ed. Atlanta, GA: Arthritis Foundation, 1997.

Kubler-Ross, E. *On Death and Dying.* New York, NY: Macmillan Publishing Co., 1981.

Leeds, Dorothy, with Jon M. Strauss, MD. *Smart Questions to Ask Your Doctor.* New York, NY: Harper Collins, 1992.

Lorig, RN, DrPH, Kate and James F. Fries, MD. *The Arthritis Helpbook: A Tested Self-Management Program for Coping with Arthritis and Fibromyalgia.* Reading, MA: Addison-Wesley Publishing Co., 1995.

Lorig, Kate, H. Holman, D. Sobel, D. Laurent, V. L. Gonzalez, and M. Minor. *Living a Healthy Life with Chronic Conditions.* Palo Alto, CA: Bull Publishing, 1994.

Lupus Foundation. *Successful Living with Chronic Illness.* Dubuque, IA: Kendall-Hunt Publishing Co., 1994.

McCall, MD, Timothy B. *Examining Your Doctor: A Patient's Guide to Avoiding Harmful Medical Care.* New York, NY: Carol Publishing Group, 1995.

Pellegrino, MD, Mark. *The Fibromyalgia Survivor.* Columbus, OH: Anadem Publishing Inc., 1995.

Pellegrino, MD, Mark. *Fibromyalgia: Managing the Pain.* Columbus, OH: Anadem Publishing Inc., 1993.

Pellegrino, MD, Mark. *Laugh at Your Muscles.* Columbus, OH: Anadem Publishing Inc., 1993.

Schneider, J. *Stress, Loss and Grief: Understanding Their Origins and Growth Potential.* Rockville, MD: Aspen Systems Corporation, 1984.

Booklets

Coping with Fibromyalgia (1991)— Booklet by Beth Ediger, a person with fibromyalgia, about symptoms, research, treatments, effects on social life, and coping. The "little red book" of basic information. 38 pages. To order: Fibromyalgia Association of Texas, 5650 Forest Lane, Dallas, TX 75230, 972/271-5085. Cost: $6.95.

Fibromyalgia in Young People: A Guide for Parents — This 60-page booklet is full of information and advice for parents of young people with fibromyalgia. To order: Fibromyalgia Network, P.O. Box 31750, Tucson, AZ 85751-1750, 800/853-2929. Cost: $10.

Fibromyalgia: Fighting Back (1992) — Booklet by Bev Spencer, a person with fibromyalgia, about taking charge of fibromyalgia, talking to doctors, exercising, sleeping better, reducing stress, and other positive steps for coping with fibromyalgia. 40 pages. To order: LRH Publications, Box 8, Station Q, Toronto, ON M4T 2L7, Canada, 416/324-8809. Cost: $6.95.

The Fibromyalgia Syndrome (1991) — Booklet by Mary Anne Saathoff, RN, Executive Director of the Fibromyalgia Alliance of America. Written for the public. Includes symptoms, diagnosis, history, causes, and treatment. 22 pages. To order: Fibromyalgia Alliance of America, P.O. Box 21990, Columbus, OH 43221-0900, 614/457-4222. Cost: $4.

The Fibromyalgia Syndrome (**1993**) — Technical information for health-care providers from the *Primer on the Rheumatic Diseases* published by the Arthritis Foundation. To order the Primer: Arthritis Foundation, P.O. Box 6996, Alpharetta, GA 30239, 800/207-8633. Cost: $25.

Getting the Most Out of Your Meds (1995) — This 28-page booklet provides a review of the drugs available for fibromyalgia and chronic fatigue syndrome treatment, an explanation of why they might work, and tips on how patients may reap the most benefits from them. Also discussed are medications commonly prescribed for TMJ, irritable bowel syndrome, and chronic headaches. To order: Fibromyalgia Network, P.O. Box 31750, Tucson, AZ 85751-1750, 800/853-2929. Cost: $7.

Brochures

Aspirin and Other NSAIDs (1996) — This 16-page brochure discusses aspirin and other nonsteroidal anti-inflammatory drugs, including dosage, side effects, and important tips to remember when taking them. To order one copy: Arthritis Foundation, 1330 W. Peachtree St., Atlanta, GA 30309, 800/283-7800. To order copies in multiples of 50: P.O. Box 6996, Alpharetta, GA 30329, 800/207-8633.

Choosing a Health Plan (1996) — This 28-page booklet will help you learn what managed care is, what types of health-care plans are available, and how to choose one that best meets your needs. To order one copy: Arthritis Foundation, 1330 West Peachtree St., Atlanta, GA 30309, 800/283-7800. To order copies in multiples of 50: P.O. Box 6996, Alpharetta, GA 30329, 800/207-8633. Cost: Single copies are free.

Coping with Depression in a Chronic Illness (1995) — This 14-page brochure is a helpful primer on coping with and accepting change. To order: Michigan Lupus Foundation, 26202 Harper Ave., St. Clair Shores, MI 48081, 810/775-8310. Cost: $3.50 plus $1.50 shipping/handling.

The Drug Guide (1995) — Originally featured in the July/August issue of *Arthritis Today*, this 16-page guide will educate you about the drugs you take for your arthritis. To order one copy: Arthritis Foundation, 1330 W. Peachtree St., Atlanta, GA 30309, 800/283-7800. To order copies in multiples of 50: P.O. Box 6996, Alpharetta, GA 30329, 800/207-8633.

Fibromyalgia (rev. 1996) — Brochure distributed by Arthritis Foundation describing symptoms and signs, diagnosis, causes, treatment, and coping with fibromyalgia. 12 pages. To order one copy: Arthritis Foundation, 1330 W. Peachtree St., Atlanta, GA 30309, 800/283-7800. To order copies in multiples of 50: P.O. Box 6996, Alpharetta, GA 30329, 800/207-8633.

Fibromyalgia Syndrome: A Primer (1996) — Brochure by Jon Russell, MD, PhD, describing prevalence, symptoms, diagnosis, and treatment. Distributed by Dr. Russell at the University of Texas Health Science Center. To order: The University of Texas Health Science Center, 7703 Floyd Curl Dr., San Antonio, TX 78284-7874. Cost: Single copies are free.

Fibromyalgia Syndrome: An Informational Guide for Fibromyalgia Patients, their Families, Friends and Employers (1994) — Informational brochure written by Robert Bennett, MD, regarding symptoms, diagnosis, treatment, support groups, research, and information resources. To order: National Fibromyalgia Research Association, Inc., P.O. Box 500, Salem, OR 97308. Cost: Single copies are free, with business-size SASE.

Managing Your Activities (1996) — This 16-page brochure describes ways to reduce the stress on joints affected by arthritis and related conditions while you're doing ordinary tasks. To order one copy: Arthritis Foundation, 1330 West Peachtree St., Atlanta, GA 30309, 800/283-7800. To order copies in multiples of 50: P.O. Box 6996, Alpharetta, GA 30329, 800/207-8633.

Managing Your Fatigue (1996) — This 16-page brochure gives basic information about what fatigue is and tips on how you can learn to manage it. To order one copy: Arthritis Foundation, 1330 West Peachtree St., Atlanta, GA 30309, 800/283-7800. To order copies in multiples of 50: P.O. Box 6996, Alpharetta, GA 30329, 800/207-8633.

Managing Your Health Care (1996) — This 16-page brochure offers basic information about working with the members of your health-care team. To order one copy: Arthritis Foundation, 1330 West Peachtree St., Atlanta, GA 30309, 800/283-7800. To order copies in multiples of 50: P.O. Box 6996, Alpharetta, GA 30329, 800/207-8633.

Managing Your Pain (1996) — This brochure suggests different ways that people with arthritis and related conditions can better manage their pain. You may want to read the entire brochure or only the sections that apply to you. 28 pages. To order one copy: Arthritis Foundation, 1330 West Peachtree St., Atlanta, GA 30309, 800/283-7800. To order copies in multiples of 50: P.O. Box 6996, Alpharetta, GA 30329, 800/207-8633.

Managing Your Stress (1996) — This brochure offers basic information about what causes stress and tips on how you can learn to manage it. 16 pages. To order one copy: Arthritis Foundation, 1330 West Peachtree St., Atlanta, GA 30309, 800/283-7800. To order more than one copy: P.O. Box 6996, Alpharetta, GA 30329, 800/207-8633.

NIAMS Information Packet (1993) — Packet of information on fibromyalgia distributed by National Institute of Arthritis and Musculoskeletal and Skin Diseases (NIAMS) containing list of organizations concerned with fibromyalgia, a glossary, the American College of Rheumatology's Fact Sheet, and several articles on fibromyalgia written by authorities in the field. To order: NAMSIC (National Arthritis, Musculoskeletal and Skin Diseases Information Clearinghouse), One AMS Circle, Bethesda, MD, 20892-3675, 301/495-4484. Publication No. AR-91. Cost: Free.

Newsletters

Bulletin on the Rheumatic Diseases — Published eight times a year by the Arthritis Foundation, this eight-page newsletter summarizes current rheumatology research and raises compelling questions about the future of caring for people with rheumatic diseases. Written for non-rheumatology health-care providers. To order: Arthritis Foundation, 1330 West Peachtree St., Atlanta, GA 30309. Cost: Free.

Fibromyalgia Network — National quarterly newsletter with information about coping, disability issues, insurance claims, treatment options, etc. To order: Fibromyalgia Network, P.O. Box 31750, Tucson, AZ 85751-1750, 502/290-5508 or 800/853-2929. Cost: $19 (U.S.) or $21 (Canada) per year. Back issues available.

The Fibromyalgia Times — National newsletter (membership benefit) of the Fibromyalgia Alliance of America. Quarterly, 20-page newsletter contains articles by health professionals on chronic pain, treatment, psychological issues, national research, government issues, and questions and answers. To order: Fibromyalgia Alliance of America, P.O. Box 21990, Columbus, OH 43221-0990, 614/457-4222. Cost: $25 per year membership.

Journal of Musculoskeletal Pain — Peer-reviewed medical journal containing FMS scientific abstract information. Appropriate for the public as well as medical professionals. Quarterly publication. To order: Haworth Medical Press, 10 Alice St., Binghamton, NY 13904, 800/342-9678. Email address: getinfo@blue.spectra.net. Cost: $36 (individual) annual subscription.

Video and Audiocassettes

Mid-Atlantic Conference on Fibromyalgia Treatment (1996) — Proceedings of the September 1996 conference are available on audiocassette. Set of six 90-minute audiocassettes. To order: Fibromyalgia Association of Greater Washington, D.C. (FMAGW), Suite 500, 12210 Fairfax Towne Center, Fairfax, VA 22033, 703/790-2324. Cost: $72 for general public.

Fibromyalgia - One Day Seminar (1993, 1994) — Audiotapes of day-long forums sponsored by the Arthritis Foundation Rocky Mountain Chapter. Includes sessions by rheumatologists, neurologists, psychiatrists, psychologists, and occupational therapists. To order: Arthritis Foundation, Rocky Mountain Chapter, 2280 South Albion St., Denver, CO 80222-4906, 303/756-8622 or call 800/475-6447 for an order blank. Website: http://www.arthritis.org. Cost: $6 each or $5 each for three or more.

What's New in Fibromyalgia - Third National Seminar (1994) — Series of seven videos and 13 audiotapes about basic research, growth hormone factors, exercise, long-term outcomes, post-traumatic fibromyalgia, legal issues, coping with fibromyalgia, and "ask the experts." Some information too technical for average audience, although much useful information is covered. For more information contact Fibromyalgia Alliance of America, P.O. Box 21990, Columbus, OH 43221-0990, 614/457-4222. Cost: $30 per video or $165 for complete set of seven videos; $15 for set of two audiotapes or $75 for complete set of 13.

Fibromyalgia: The Invisible Pain (1991) — Videotape that describes fibromyalgia, its symptoms, and treatment. Several people with fibromyalgia relate what it is like to have the disease and how they cope. 15 minutes. To order: Arthritis Foundation, Southern California Chapter, 4311 Wilshire Blvd., Suite 503, Los Angeles, CA 90010, 213/954-5750. Cost: $15.

Fibromyalgia Workshop on Legal and Disability Issues (1993) — Videotape which includes sessions provided by physicians on fibromyalgia diagnosis, treatment, and medications, and by legal experts on their needs for medical documentation for disability and how to obtain SSDI and worker's compensation. 122 minutes. To order: Arthritis Foundation Southern California Chapter, 4311 Wilshire Blvd., Suite 503, Los Angeles, CA 90010, 213/954-5750. Cost: Available for free loan.

Fibromyalgia Stretching Video — by Sharon R. Clark, PhD, FNP. To order: National Fibromyalgia Research Association, P.O. Box 500, Salem, OR 97308, 503/228-3217. Cost: $19.95. Add $5 shipping and handling for each tape. Allow four to six weeks for delivery.

Good Moves for Every Body exercise video — Includes range-of-motion, muscle- strengthening, and endurance-building exercise. View on the website: http://www.hsc. missouri.edu/shrp/goodmove. To order: Multipurpose Arthritis Center, Attention: Exercise Video, FOLK Hall 22, University of Missouri, Columbia, MO, 65212, 573/882-8097. Cost: $30, shipping included.

ROM Dance — Each of these three ROM dance videotapes includes step-by-step instructions that clearly show how to do a series of gentle range-of-motion exercises. It is accompanied by soothing music and a pleasant verse. The videos also include a guided relaxation session to enhance your body awareness and stir your imagination with healthful images. The three videotapes include: the *ROM Dance in Sunlight* (original version of the ROM Dance, using images of sunlight, warm water, and friendship); the *ROM Dance in Moonlight* (adapted for people with sunlight sensitivity, using images of moonlight, water, and friendship); and the *ROM Dance: Seated Version* (adapted for those with difficulty standing or who use wheelchairs; tape also includes the *ROM Dance in Sunlight*). To order: The ROM Dance, P.O. Box 3332, Madison, WI 53704-0332, 800/488-4940. Cost: $24.95 per video (shipping and handling additional). Discounts available for bulk orders.

Relaxation Audiocassettes — The following audiocassettes may be helpful if used in conjunction with the activities in Chapter 8.

Bull Publishing Co., P.O. Box 208, Palo Alto, CA 94302-0208, 800/676-2855.

Tape 1: Arthritis Self-Management Participant's Tape

Designed to be used with Arthritis Self-Help Course and includes four 15-minute relaxation exercises with background music and the voice of Catherine Regan, PhD.

1-Progressive Muscle Relaxation helps you achieve deep muscular relaxation and releases tension; it also quiets the mind and emotions.

2-Guided Imagery: A Walk in the Country uses the imagination to travel to a pleasant place and time, helping you to achieve total relaxation and heightened self-awareness.

3-Autogenic Relaxation enhances the mind's ability to initiate desired physical responses.

4-Visualization assists you in using your mind to recall past successes and achieve future goals.

Tape 2: Arthritis Self-Management Group Leader's Tape

Designed to be used with Arthritis Self-Help Course and includes condensed versions of the progressive muscle relaxation, guided imagery, and visualization exercises. Also included is a specific exercise in using visualization to achieve your goals, designed to be used at the end of each class session in conjunction with contracting.

To order: Cost: $10 each (shipping and handling not included). Bulk orders: 1-9 tapes, $10 each; 10-49 tapes, $8 each; 50-499 tapes, $7.50 each; 500 tapes, $7 each (shipping and handling not included).

Whole Person Associates, 210 West Michigan St., Duluth, MN 55802-1908, 800/247-6789.

Over 20 different tapes are available on deep breathing, progressive muscle relaxation, autogenic relaxation, meditation, guided imagery, and visualization. Here's a sampling:

Tape 1: Take a Deep Breath.
> Side A: Breathing for Relaxation and Health
> Side B: The Magic Ball

Tape 2: Relax. . . Let go . . . Relax
> Side A: Revitalization
> Side B: Relaxation

Tape 3: Stress Release
> Side A: Quick Tension Relaxers
> Side B: Progressive Relaxation.

To order: Cost: $11.95 each (plus shipping and handling). Call 800/247-6789 for a catalog.

Suggested Reading from Professional Journals

Bengtsson, A., K. G. Henriksson, L. Jorfeldt, B. Kagedal, C. Lenmarken, and F. Lindstrom. "Primary Fibromyalgia. A Clinical and Laboratory Study of 55 Patients." *Scandinavian Journal of Rheumatology,* 1986; 15:340-7.

Bengtsson, A., K. G. Henriksson, and J. Larsson. "Reduced High-Energy Phosphate Levels in the Painful Muscles of Patients with Primary Fibromyalgia." *Arthritis & Rheumatism,* 1986; 29:817-21.

Bennett, R. M., S. R. Clark, S. M. Campbell, and C. S. Burckhardt. "Somatomedin-C Levels in Patients with the Fibromyalgia Syndrome: a Possible Link Between Sleep and Muscle Pain." *Arthritis & Rheumatism,* 1992: 35, 1113-6.

Bennett, R. M. "Etiology of the Fibromyalgia Syndrome: a Contemporary Hypothesis." *Internal Medicine Specialist* 1990; 11:48-61.

Bennett, R. M. "The Origin of Myopain: An Integrated Hypothesis of Focal Muscle Changes and Sleep Disturbance in Patients with the Fibromyalgia Syndrome." *Journal of Musculoskeletal Pain,* 1993.

Burckhardt, C. S., S. R. Clark, and R. M. Bennett. "Fibromyalgia and Quality of Life: a Comparative Analysis." *Journal of Rheumatology,* 1993: 20:475-9.

Burckhardt, C. S., S. R. Clark, and R. M. Bennett. "The Fibromyalgia Impact Questionnaire: Development and Validation." *Journal of Rheumatology,* 1991; 18:728-33.

Callahan, L. F., and T. Pincus. "A Clue From a Self-Report Questionnaire to Distinguish Rheumatoid Arthritis from Noninflammatory Diffuse Musculoskeletal Pain." The P-VAS:D-ADL ratio. *Arthritis and Rheumatism,* 1990; 33:1317-22.

Cathey, M. A., F. Wolfe, S. M. Kleinheksel, and D. J. Hawley. "Socioeconomic Impact of Fibrositis. A Study of 81 Patients with Primary Fibrositis." *American Journal of Medicine,* 1986; 81:78-84.

Cathey, M. A., F. Wolfe, S. M. Kleinheksel, et al. "Functional Ability and Work Status in Patients with Fibromyalgia." *Arthritis Care and Research,* 1988; 1:85-98.

Cathey, M. A., F. Wolfe, F. K. Roberts, et al. "Demographics Work Disability, Service Utilization and Treatment Characteristics of 620 Fibromyalgia Patients in Rheumatologic Practice (abstract)." *Arthritis and Rheumatism,* 1990; 33:S10.

Clark, S. R., C. S. Burckhardt, S. Campbell, C. O'Reilly, and R. M. Bennett. "Fitness Characteristics and perceived Exertion in Women with Fibromyalgia." *Journal of Musculoskeletal Pain, 1993.*

Cuneo, R. C., F. Salomon, G. A. McGauley, and P. H. Sönksen. "Psychological Well-Being before and after Growth Hormone Treatment in Adults with Growth Hormone Deficiency." *Hormone Research,* 1990; (suppl 4) 33:52-4.

Cuneo, R. C., F. Salomon, C. M. Wiles, R. Hesp, and P. H. Sönksen. "Growth Hormone Treatment in Growth Hormone-Deficient Adults. Effects on Exercise Performance." *Journal of Applied Physiology,* 1991; 70:695-700.

Cuneo, R. C., F. Salomon, C. M. Wiles, and P. H. Sönksen. "Skeletal Muscle Performance in Adults with Growth Hormone Deficiency." *Hormone Research,* 1990; (suppl 4) 33:55-60.

Cuneo, R. C., F. Salomon, P. Wilmhurst, et al. "Cardiovascular Effects of Growth Hormone Treatment in Growth-Hormone Deficient Adults: Stimulation of the Renin-Aldosterone System." *Clinical Science* 1991; 81:587-92.

Diagnostic and Statistical Manual of Mental Disorders. Washington: American Psychiatric Association. 1987.

Elert, J. E., S. B. Rantapää Dahlquist, K. Henriksson-Larsen, and B. Gerdle. "Increased EMG Activity during Short Pauses in Patients with Primary Fibromyalgia." *Scandinavian Journal of Rheumatology,* 1989; 18:321-3.

Fryburg, D. A., R. J. Louard, K. E. Gerow, R. A. Gelfand, and E. J. Barrett. "Growth Hormone Stimulates Skeletal Muscle Protein Synthesis and Antagonizes Insulin's Antiproteolytic Action in Humans." *Diabetes,* 1992; 41:424-9.

Greenfield, S., M. A. Fitzcharles, and J. M. Esdaile. "Reactive Fibromyalgia Syndrome." *Arthritis and Rheumatism,* 1992; 35:678-81.

Guest, G. H., and P. D. Drummond. "Effects of Compensation on Emotional State and Disability in Chronic Back Pain." *Pain* 1992; 48:125-30.

Hawley, D. J., and F. Wolfe. "Pain, Disability and Pain/Disability Relationships in Seven Rheumatic Disorders: A Study of 1,522 Patients." *Journal of Rheumatology,* 1991; 18:1552-7.

Henriksson, C., I. Gundmark, A. Bengtsson, and A. C. Ek. "Living with Fibromyalgia. Consequences for Everyday Life." *Clinical Journal of Pain* 1992; 8:138-44.

Henriksson, K. G., and A. Bengtsson. "Muscular Changes in Fibromyalgia and Their Significance in Diagnosis." *Advances in Pain Research* 1990; 17:259-67.

Holl, R. W., M. L. Hartman, J. D. Veldhuis, W. M. Taylor, and M. O. Thorner. "Thirty-Second Sampling of Plasma Growth Hormone in Man: Correlation with Sleep Stages." *Journal of Clinical Endocrinology and Metabolism,* 1991; 72:854-61.

Jacobsen, S., and B. Danneskiold-Samsoe. "Dynamic Muscular Endurance in Primary Fibromyalgia Compared with Chronic Myofascial Pain Syndrome." *Archives of Physical Medicine and Rehabilitation,* 1992; 72:170-3.

Jacobsen, S. G. Wildschiodtz, and B. Danneskiold-Samsoe. "Isokinetic and Isometric Muscle Strength Combined with Transcutaneous Electrical Muscle Strength Stimulation in Primary Fibromyalgia Syndrome." *Journal of Rheumatology,* 1991; 18:1390-3.

Littlejohn, G. "Fibrositis/Fibromyalgia Syndrome in the Workplace." *Rheumatic Disease Clinics of North America,* 1989; 15:45-60.

Littlejohn, G. "Medicolegal Aspects of Fibrositis Syndrome." *Journal of Rheumatology,* 1989; (suppl 19) 16:167-73.

Lund, N., A. Bengtsson, and P. Thorborg. "Muscle Tissue Oxygen Pressure in Primary Fibromyalgia." *Scandinavian Journal of Rheumatology,* 1986; 15:165-73.

Lundeberg, S., M. Belfrage, J. Wernerman, A. Von der Decken, S. Thunell, and E. Vinnars. "Growth Hormone Improves Muscle Protein

"Metabolism and Whole Body Nitrogen Economy in Man During a Hyponitrogenous Diet." *Metabolism* 1991; 40:315-22.

McCain, G. A., R. Cameron, and J. C. Kennedy. "The Problem of Longterm Disability Payments and Litigation in Primary Fibromyalgia: The Canadian perspective." *Journal of Rheumatology,* 1989; (suppl 19) 16:175-6.

McGauley, G.A., R. C. Cuneo, F. Salomon, and P. H. Sönksen. "Psychological Well Being before and after Growth Hormone Treatment in Adults with Growth Hormone Deficiency." *Hormone Research,* 1990; (suppl 4) 33:52-4.

Moldofsky, H., MTH Won, and F. A. Lue. "Litigation, Sleep Symptoms and Disabilities in Postaccident Pain (Fibromyalgia)." *Journal of Rheumatology,* 1993; 20:1935-40.

Moldofsky, H. "Sleep and Fibrositis Syndrome." *Rheumatic Disease Clinics of North America,* 1989; 15:91-103.

Prince, M. "Association Neuroses: A Study of the Pathology of Hysterical Joint Affections, Neurasthenia and Allied Forms of Neuro-Mimesis." *Journal of Nervous and Mental Disease,* 1981; 18:257-82.

Radanov, B. P., G. Di Stefano, A. Schnidrig, and P. Ballinari. "Role of Psychosocial Stress in Recovery from Common Whiplash." *Lancet,* 1991; 388:712-5.

Romano, T. J. "Clinical Experiences with Post-Traumatic Fibromyalgia Syndrome." *West Virginia Medical Journal,* 1990; 86:198-202.

Russell, MD, PhD, I. J., "Fibromyalgia Syndrome: Approaches to Management." *Bulletin on the Rheumatic Diseases, 1996; 45(3):1-40.*

Russell, I. J., J. E. Michalek, G. A. Vipraio, E. M. Fletcher, M. A. Javors, and C. A. Bowden. "Platelet 3H-Imipramine Uptake Receptor Density and Serum Serotonin Levels in Patients with Fibromyalgia/Fibrositis Syndrome." *Journal of Rheumatology,* 1992; 19:104-9.

Russell, I. J., H. Vaeroy, M. Javors, and F. Nyberg. "Cerebrospinal Fluid Biogenic Amine Metabolites in Fibromyalgia/Fibrositis Syndrome and Rheumatoid Arthritis." *Arthritis and Rheumatism,* 1992; 35:550-6.

Rutherford, O. M., D. A. Jones, J. M. Round, C. R. Buchanan, and M. A. Preece. "Changes in Skeletal Muscle and Body Composition after Discontinuation of Growth Hormone Treatment in Growth Hormone Deficient Young Adults." *Clinical Endocrinology (Oxford),* 1991; 34:469-75.

Vaeroy, H., R. Helle, O. Forre, E. Kass, and L. Terenius. "Elevated CSF Levels of Substance P and High Incidence of Raynaud Phenomenon in Patients with Fibromyalgia: New Features for Diagnosis." *Pain,* 1988; 32:21-6.

Wolfe, F., H. A. Smythe, and M. B .Yunus, et al. "The American College of Rheumatology 1990 Criteria for the Classification of Fibromyalgia: Report of the Multicenter Criteria Committee." *Arthritis and Rheumatism,* 1990; 33:160-72.

Yunus, M. B., J. W. Dailey, J. C. Aldag, A. T. Masi, and P. C. Jobe. "Plasma Tryptophan and Other Amino Acids in Primary Fibromyalgia: A Controlled Study." *Journal of Rheumatology,* 1992; 19:90-4.

Suggested Reading from Arthritis Today magazine

To order a free copy of any of these articles: Arthritis Foundation, 1330 West Peachtree St., Atlanta, GA 30309, 800/283-7800.

"Arthritis 101" (1995) — Originally featured in the May-June issue, this article offers answers to 21 of your basic questions.

"Craving a Cure" (1996) — Article from May-June issue discussing the connection between food and arthritis symptoms.

"The Drug Guide" (1995) — Originally featured in the July-August issue. This guide will educate you about the drugs you take for your arthritis.

"Fibromyalgia" (1993) — Article from September-October issue describing treatment, management, and coping skills for fibromyalgia syndrome.

"The Point of Pain" (1995) — Article from November-December issue discusses the messenger that is chronic pain.

"The Voluntary Reflex" (1996) — Article from May-June issue discussing the risks involved in volunteering for arthritis research.

Organizations

American College of Rheumatology
60 Executive Park South, Suite 150
Atlanta, GA 30329
404/633-3777

Arthritis Foundation
1330 West Peachtree St.
Atlanta, GA 30309
404/872-7100
800/283-7800

Fibromyalgia Alliance of America
P.O. Box 21990
Columbus, OH 43221-0990
614/457-4222

Fibromyalgia Association of Greater Washington, D.C. (FMAGW)
Suite 500
12210 Fairfax Towne Center
Fairfax, VA 22033
703/790-2324

Fibromyalgia Association of Texas
3810 Keele Dr.
Garland, TX 75041
972/271-5085

Fibromyalgia Network
P.O. Box 31750
Tuscon, AZ 85751-1750
502/290-5508
800/853-2929

Job Accommodations Network
West Virginia University
P.O. Box 6080
Morgantown, WV 26506-6080
website: http://janweb.icdi.wvu.edu
800/526-7234

National Arthritis, Musculoskeletal and Skin Diseases Information
Clearinghouse (NAMSIC)
One AMS Circle
Bethesda, MD 20892-3675
301/495-4484

National Council on Independent Living
2111 Wilson Blvd., Ste. 405
Arlington, VA 22201
703/525-3406

National Fibromyalgia Research Association Inc.
P.O. Box 500
Salem, OR 97308

National Organization for Rare Disorders (NORD)
P.O. Box 8923
New Fairfield, CT 06812-8923
website: http://www.nord-rdb.com/~orphan
800/447-6673

Social Security Disability Advocates Inc.
23930 Michigan Ave.
Dearborn, MI 48124
800/628-2887

About the Arthritis Foundation

The Arthritis Foundation is the source of help and hope for nearly 40 million Americans who have arthritis and related diseases and conditions. Founded in 1948, the Arthritis Foundation is the only national, voluntary health organization that works for all people affected by any of the more than 100 forms of arthritis or related diseases. Volunteers in chapters nationwide help to support research, professional, and community education programs, services for people with arthritis, government advocacy, and fund-raising activities.

The American Juvenile Arthritis Organization (AJAO) is composed of children, parents, teachers, and others concerned specifically about juvenile arthritis and related diseases and conditions. A council of the Arthritis Foundation, AJAO focuses its efforts on the problems related to arthritis in children.

The focus of the Arthritis Foundation is twofold: to support research to find the cure for and prevention of arthritis, and to improve the quality of life for those affected by arthritis. Public contributions enable the Arthritis Foundation to fulfill this mission—in fact, at least 80 cents of every dollar donated to the Arthritis Foundation serves to directly fund research and program services.

The Arthritis Foundation Helps

Fibromyalgia — one of the more than 100 rheumatic diseases and conditions related to arthritis — doesn't have to rob you of the activities you enjoy most. While research holds the key to future cures or preventions for fibromyalgia and other arthritis-related conditions, equally important is improving your quality of life.

Your local chapter of the Arthritis Foundation has printed information, a self-help course designed for people with fibromyalgia, exercise classes, and other services to put you in charge of your fibromyalgia. The Arthritis Foundation has more than 150 local offices across the United States. To find the office near you, and to determine which of the following resources are available through your nearest chapter, call 800/283-7800.

Medical and Self-Care Programs

1. Physician referral — Most Arthritis Foundation chapters have a list of doctors in your area who specialize in the evaluation and treatment of arthritis and arthritis-related conditions such as fibromyalgia.

2. Exercise programs — Recreational in nature, these are developed, coordinated, and sponsored by the Arthritis Foundation. All have specially trained instructors. They include:

- **Joint Efforts** — This movement program teaches gentle, undemanding movement exercises for people with arthritis and related conditions, including those who use walkers and wheelchairs. Joint Efforts is designed to encourage movement and socialization among older adults and to help decrease pain, stiffness, and depression.

- **PACE® (People with Arthritis Can Exercise)** — PACE® is an exercise program that uses gentle activities to help increase joint flexibility, range of motion, and stamina, and to help maintain muscle strength. Two videotapes showing basic and advanced levels of the program are available from your local chapter for preview or for practice at home. Cost: $19.50 each (nonmembers), $15.75 (members). Shipping and handling not included. To order the videos, call 800/933-0032.

- **Arthritis Foundation Aquatic Program** — Originally co-developed by the YMCA and the Arthritis Foundation, this water exercise program helps relieve the strain on muscles and joints for people with arthritis and related conditions.

- **PEP (Pool Exercise Program)** — This videotape shows how to exercise on your own. $19.50 (nonmembers), $15.75 (members). Shipping and handling not included. To order the video, call 800/933-0032.

- **FIT (Fibromyalgia Interval Training)** — This videotape is an advanced aquatic program designed to help manage pain, stiffness, and fatigue. Features exercises in deep and shallow water in an interval training format. Cost: $29.99 (nonmembers), $22.50 (members). Shipping and handling not included. To order the video, call 800/933-0032.

Educational and/or Emotional Support Groups

For more information on the following groups, call your local Arthritis Foundation chapter. To find a chapter near you, call 800/283-7800.

1. Arthritis Foundation Support and Education Groups — These are mutual-support groups that provide opportunities for discussion and problem solving. They are usually formed by people with arthritis and related conditions and/or their family members who wish to meet with their peers for mutual assistance in satisfying common needs and in overcoming problems related to arthritis.

2. Classes/Courses — Formal group meetings help you gain the knowledge, skills, and confidence you need to actively manage your conditions. Courses focus on proper exercises, medications, relaxation techniques, pain management, dealing with depression, nutrition, non-traditional treatments, and doctor-patient relations. Courses on arthritis, fibromyalgia and lupus are available.

Fibromyalgia Self-Help Course — This seven-week educational program is designed specifically to teach people with fibromyalgia how to take a more active role in their health care. The course provides information, skills, and support to people with fibromyalgia and their families to help them better cope with the condition.

Reliable Information at Your Fingertips

1. Information hot line — The Arthritis Foundation is *the* expert on arthritis and related conditions and is only a phone call away. Call toll free at 800/283-7800 for automated information on arthritis 24 hours a day. Trained volunteers and staff are also available at your local Arthritis Foundation chapter to answer your questions or send you a list of physicians in your area who specialize in arthritis and related conditions.

2. Arthritis Foundation Web site — Information about arthritis and related conditions is available 24 hours a day to Internet users via the Arthritis Foundation's site on the World Wide Web. The address for the web site is http://www.arthritis.org.

3. Publications — A number of publications are available to educate you about important considerations such as medications, exercise, diet, pain management, and stress management, to name a few.

- **Books** — Self-help books are available from the Arthritis Foundation to help you learn more about your condition and how to manage it. Check your local bookstores, your local Arthritis Foundation chapter, or order a book through the Arthritis Foundation by calling 800/207-8633.

- **Booklets** — More than 60 booklets and brochures provide information on the many arthritis-related diseases and conditions, medications, how to work with your doctor, and how to care for yourself. Single copies are available free of charge. Call 800/283-7800 for a free listing of booklets on arthritis.
- *Arthritis Today* — The award-winning bimonthly magazine *Arthritis Today* gives you the latest information on research, new treatments, and tips from experts and readers to help you manage arthritis and related conditions. Each issue also brings you information on fibromyalgia, as well as a variety of helpful and interesting articles covering diet and nutrition, tips for traveling, and ways you can make your life with arthritis and musculoskeletal problems easier and more rewarding. A one-year subscription to *Arthritis Today* is yours free when you become a member of the Arthritis Foundation. Annual membership is $20 and helps fund research to find cures for arthritis. Call 800/933-0032 for membership and subscription information.

4. Speakers' bureau — Lay and professional volunteers conduct educational presentations to various groups. To schedule a speaker for your group, call your local Arthritis Foundation chapter.

5. Public forums — Educational programs are presented to your community on various requested topics. Call the Arthritis Foundation chapter in your area for more information.

6. Professional publications — A number of professional education materials on arthritis and related conditions geared to the health-care professional are available through the Arthritis Foundation. These materials, including the *Bulletin on the Rheumatic Diseases* newsletter which is published eight times a year, and the 356-page *Primer on the Rheumatic Diseases* which is published every five years, are available by calling 404/872-7100.

7. Audiovisual libraries — Available either on loan or for purchase, a number of audio- and videocassettes cover a variety of topics from exercise to relaxation. Call the chapter in your area for a listing of titles, prices, and availabilities.

Remember the Arthritis Foundation in Your Will

Planned giving is an important part of fulfilling the Arthritis Foundation's mission to support arthritis research and improve the quality of life for those affected by arthritis. The Arthritis Foundation offers a wide variety of gift planning options — gifts of cash, appreciated assets, gifts by will or living trust, naming the Arthritis Foundation as beneficiary of your life insurance, individual retirement account (IRA), pension, 401(k), or other retirement savings plan.

It is our hope that you decide to include a gift to the Arthritis Foundation in your will. Your greatest benefit in assisting the Arthritis Foundation will be the personal satisfaction of making a difference in the struggle against arthritis. For more information on giving opportunities, call the planned giving department at 404/872-7100.

Arthritis Foundation
1330 W. Peachtree St.
Atlanta, GA 30309
404-872-7100
http://www.arthritis.org

Notes

Notes

Notes